PHONETIC SCIENCE FOR CLINICAL PRACTICE

A Transcription and Application Workbook

SECOND EDITION

PHONETIC SCIENCE FOR CLINICAL PRACTICE

A Transcription and Application Workbook

SECOND EDITION

Kathy J. Jakielski, PhD, CCC-SLP, ASHA Fellow
Christina E. Gildersleeve-Neumann, PhD, CCC-SLP, ASHA Fellow

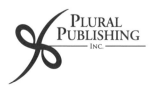

PLURAL
PUBLISHING
INC.

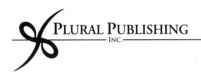

9177 Aero Drive, Suite B
San Diego, CA 92123

email: information@pluralpublishing.com
website: https://www.pluralpublishing.com

Typeset in 11/14 Stone Informal by Flanagan's Publishing Services, Inc.
Printed in the United States of America by Sheridan Saline

Library of Congress Cataloging-in-Publication Data:
ISBN-13: 978-1-63550-407-1
ISBN-10: 1-63550-407-4

NOTICE TO THE USER
Care has been taken to confirm the accuracy of the indications, procedures, drug dosages, and diagnosis and remediation protocols presented in this book and to ensure that they conform to the practices of the general medical and health services communities. However, the authors, editors, and publisher are not responsible for errors or omissions or for any consequences from application of the information in this book and make no warranty, expressed or implied, with respect to the currency, completeness, or accuracy of the contents of the publication. The diagnostic and remediation protocols and the medications described do not necessarily have specific approval by the Food and Drug administration for use in the disorders and/or diseases and dosages for which they are recommended. Application of this information in a particular situation remains the professional responsibility of the practitioner. Because standards of practice and usage change, it is the responsibility of the practitioner to keep abreast of revised recommendations, dosages, and procedures.

CONTENTS

There is a lot to learn in a phonetics course. To understand the science and the clinical application of phonetics, extensive practice is essential. This workbook, a companion to *Phonetic Science for Clinical Practice, Second Edition,* provides a variety of activities to promote student understanding of newly acquired concepts. It emphasizes the understanding of the science behind the practical application of phonetics and the scientific connection to hearing and speech sciences. The questions posed in this workbook tie directly to information in the textbook, allowing students to assess their understanding of concepts and to get practice transcribing speech.

How to Use This Workbook

This workbook is divided into 10 chapters. The workbook content in Chapters 1 through 9 is directly related to Chapters 1 through 9 in your textbook. These workbook chapters expand on textbook chapters in several ways. There are questions that mirror the "Did You Get It" sections of each textbook chapter, as well as other extension activities. Exercises to increase transcription skills are first introduced in Chapter 2. Transcription exercises in later chapters apply concepts covered in each chapter in the textbook. Chapter 10 is devoted exclusively to transcription practice. Transcription difficulty progresses throughout Chapter 10, with the earlier sections covering single syllable words, progressing to longer sentences. We advise completing sections of Chapter 10 as they match your level of transcription skill.

Both our textbook and our workbook present phonetics from a General American English perspective. This is a simplistic view of English and transcription and is merely a starting point for your transcription skills and phonetic science knowledge. We encourage you to apply this foundation to other dialects of English, other languages, and disordered speech.

Unless indicated otherwise, you can use broad phonemic transcription for the transcription exercises. The only exception is the indication of the allophonic [ɾ] in the answer key. Because /ɑ/ and /ɔ/ are phonemic for some GAE speakers and allophonic for other GAE speakers, the answer key shows both versions as correct. Your professor may request that you add phonetic details to your exercises or that you emphasize dialectal differences present in your community.

Multimedia Components

The workbook includes audio files for transcription practice. Words or sounds with accompanying audio files are highlighted in green. These audio files are found on the workbook's companion website.

This workbook is dedicated to our students. Your feedback over the years is at the core of these exercises and transcription sentences. We want to thank the students who helped create the exercises in this book, including Jillian Adkins, Kristina Cruz, Cara Dick, Nathan Hartleben, McKenzie Hendricks, Heather Mason, Bethany Miller, Jennifer Otwell, Evelyn Pulkowski, Micaela Quintana, and Summer Zeimetz. In particular, we would like to thank Jordan Siegel, who is the voice behind the transcription and the spectrograms, and our colleague Andy McMillin, whose expertise in recording and phonetic science was critical to the transcription components of the workbook. To David and Byron, and to Jonathan, Simona, and Elijah, thank you for always being there, for forgiving us for burying ourselves in the workbook creation, and for getting excited for us as this workbook took form.

PART

I

EXERCISES

1

INTRODUCTION TO PHONETIC SCIENCE

1–1. Branches of Phonetics

Indicate which branch of phonetics is being practiced in each scenario: articulatory, acoustic, auditory, or linguistic.

1. Determining if a *z* sound changes in spectral frequency over time by examining a speech spectrogram (a spectrogram is a visible representation of speech).

   _____

2. Determining if a child's tongue tip is raised or lowered when they produce an *s* sound by watching the child's mouth during speech production.

   _____

3. Determining if a child is transferring a sound pattern from their native language to words in their second language by examining a written transcript of the words they said.

   _____

4. Determining if a bilingual adult can differentiate between two sounds—one sound in their language and one sound in a language they do not speak.

   _____

5. Determining if the vocal folds vibrate during production of the *v* sound by feeling the laryngeal area during production.

   _____

6. Determining lip movement during production of *b* in word-final position.

   _____

7. Determining that *t* and *g* encode meaning in English because the words **"dot"** and **"dog"** are different words.

_____

8. Determining the average vocal pitch of French-speaking children.

_____

9. Determining if a grade-school child can tell the difference between sounds produced using the tip of the tongue.

_____

10. Determining that the *th* sound is meaningful in English but not in German.

_____

1–2. Phonemes and Phones

Read each pair of phrases. Place each phrase that denotes the concept of phonemes between virgules, and place the phrases that denote the concept of phones between brackets. The first pair has been done for you.

phonemes	/phonemes/
phones	[phones]
planning or production of speech sounds	_____
mental representations of speech sounds	_____
the word	_____
the word spoken	_____
the thought of producing a word	_____
the thought of a word	_____
language	_____
speech	_____
out of the mouth	_____
in the head	_____

1–3. The Continuum of Archaic to Intimate Speech Registers

A. Write the following sentences to represent **citation-form** speech.

1. Why ain'tcha goin'?

_____

2. Where ya been?

_____

3. I gotta git movin'.

_____

4. She sumpm else!

_____

5. Howdja do on the test?

_____

B. Write the following sentences to represent **casual** speech.

1. Can you believe it?

_____

2. I really want a day off.

_____

3. What did you buy?

_____

4. I would love to see you again!

_____

5. Let me help you with that.

_____

C. Fill in the following blanks. Then practice reading the paragraph aloud to someone using citation-form speech. Be clear and precise in your articulation, but avoid extreme overexaggeration. Ask your listener for feedback on your articulation. Then, think about how it felt to produce citation-form speech and to whom and in what situations would you speak using a formal or consultative register.

Hello! My name is _____ and I am very happy to meet you. I am originally from _____, and I have been living in _____ for the past _____. I am studying phonetics because _____ _____. One thing I already have learned in phonetics that I find interesting is _____.

1. Describe the feedback you received from your listener.

_____

_____

_____

_____

_____

2. Note how it felt producing formal speech.

_____

_____

_____

_____

_____

3. To whom and in what situations would you speak using a formal register?

_____

_____

_____

_____

_____

1–4. Analyzing Spoken Words: Number of Sounds and Syllables

Low Level of Difficulty

Complete the chart for the words listed.

Word	# of Sounds	# of Syllables
bat		
hip-hop		
is		
swim		
hand		
sank		
grand		
dental		
second		
analysis		
electron		
kayak		
static		
pencil		

Moderate Level of Difficulty

Complete the chart for the words listed.

Word	# of Sounds	# of Syllables
why		
gnat		
they		
six		
couch		
thumb		
known		
balloon		
ship		
amount		
right		
famous		
jumped		
knife		
success		

High Level of Difficulty

Complete the chart for the words listed.

Word	# of Sounds	# of Syllables
beauty		
extension		
refuse		
language		
spatula		
exhaust		
suggestion		
rhythm		
castle		
reputation		
studying		
vicarious		
earthquake		
ambitious		
ubiquitous		

1–5. Analyzing Spoken Words: Phonotactic Structure and Syllabicity

Low Level of Difficulty

Complete the chart for the words listed.

Word	Phonotactic Structure	Syllabicity
bat		
hip-hop		
is		
swim		
hand		
sank		
grand		
dental		
second		
analysis		
electron		
kayak		
static		
pencil		

Moderate Level of Difficulty

Complete the chart for the words listed.

Word	Phonotactic Structure	Syllabicity
why		
gnat		
they		
six		
couch		
thumb		
known		
balloon		
ship		
amount		
right		
famous		
jumped		
knife		
success		

High Level of Difficulty

Complete the chart for the words listed.

Word	Phonotactic Structure	Syllabicity
beauty		
extension		
refuse		
language		
spatula		
exhaust		
suggestion		
rhythm		
castle		
reputation		
studying		
vicarious		
earthquake		
ambitious		
ubiquitous		

1–6. Analyzing Spoken Words: Position of Consonants in Words

Complete the chart for the words listed. Leave blank any cells without data.

Word	Word-Initial Position	Word-Medial Position	Word-Final Position
bat			
is			
swim			
hand			
second			
avoid			
static			
pencil			
thumb			
balloon			
knife			
beauty			
exhaust			
suggest			
rhythm			
castle			
stringy			

1–7. Analyzing Spoken Words: Position of Consonants in Syllables

Complete the chart for the words listed. Leave blank any cells without data.

Word	Syllable-1 Initial Position	Syllable-1 Final Position	Syllable-2 Initial Position	Syllable-2 Final Position
bat				
is				
swim				
hand				
second				
avoid				
static				
pencil				
thumb				
balloon				
knife				
beauty				
exhaust				
suggest				
rhythm				
castle				
stringy				

1–8. Analyzing Spoken Words: Identifying the Stressed Syllable

For each word, indicate the syllable that is stressed. The first word has been done as an example.

Word	Stressed Syllable
dental	**first syllable**
second	
analysis	
electron	
kayak	
static	
pencil	
balloon	
amount	
famous	
jumped	
success	
beauty	
extension	
language	
spatula	
exhaust	
suggestion	
rhythm	
castle	
reputation	
studying	
vicarious	
earthquake	
ambitious	
ubiquitous	

ARTICULATORY PHONETICS: CONSONANTS

2–1. Writing Phonetic Consonant Symbols

Practice drawing each phonetic symbol several times on the line.

Name	Phonetic Symbol	Practice
eng	ŋ	
theta	θ	
ethe	ð	
esh	ʃ	
ezh	ʒ	
tesh digraph	t͡ʃ	
dezh digraph	d͡ʒ	
turned R	ɹ	

2–2. Matching Phonetic Symbols to Alphabet Letters

Match each phonetic symbol in the left-hand column with its corresponding alphabet letter(s) in the right-hand column.

1. k _____
2. ŋ _____
3. j _____
4. θ _____
5. ð _____
6. s _____
7. ʃ _____
8. t͡ʃ _____
9. d͡ʒ _____
10. ɪ _____

a. th (as in *thigh*)
b. sh
c. soft "c"
d. ch
e. ng (as in *sing*)
f. j (as in *jay*)
g. y
h. r
i. th (as in *thy*)
j. hard "c" (as in *candy*)

2–3. Identifying Voiced and Voiceless Consonant Phonemes in Isolation

Indicate if each consonant represents a sound that is voiced or voiceless.

1. p   voiced – voiceless
2. d   voiced – voiceless
3. k   voiced – voiceless
4. ɹ   voiced – voiceless
5. ʒ   voiced – voiceless
6. w   voiced – voiceless
7. f   voiced – voiceless
8. ð   voiced – voiceless
9. z   voiced – voiceless

10. h   voiced – voiceless

11. d͡ʒ   voiced – voiceless

12. l   voiced – voiceless

2–4. Identifying Voiced and Voiceless Consonant Phonemes in Words

Indicate whether each bolded consonant (or consonants) represents a phoneme that is voiced or voiceless.

  1. b as in *boo*   voiced – voiceless

  2. t as in *too*   voiced – voiceless

  3. g as in *goo*   voiced – voiceless

  4. m as in *moo*   voiced – voiceless

  5. j as in *you*   voiced – voiceless

  6. v as in *voodoo*   voiced – voiceless

  7. θ as in *through*   voiced – voiceless

  8. s as in *sue*   voiced – voiceless

  9. ʃ as in *shoe*   voiced – voiceless

10. t͡ʃ as in *chew*   voiced – voiceless

11. ɹ as in *rue*   voiced – voiceless

12. f as in *flew*   voiced – voiceless

2–5. Matching Phonetic Consonant Symbols to Articulatory Place

Match each phonetic symbol with its place of articulation.

1. z _____		a. bilabial
2. j _____		b. labiodental
3. h _____		c. interdental
4. f _____		d. alveolar
5. ð _____		e. post-alveolar
6. w _____		f. alveopalatal
7. d͡ʒ _____		g. palatal
8. ŋ _____		h. velar
9. ʃ _____		i. glottal

2–6. Matching Phonetic Consonant Symbols to Articulatory Place

Match each phonetic symbol with the appropriate place of articulation.

1. ʒ _____		a. labiodental
2. h _____		b. interdental
3. t͡ʃ _____		c. alveolar
4. ɹ _____		d. post-alveolar
5. m _____		e. alveopalatal
6. k _____		f. palatal
7. θ _____		g. velar
8. v _____		h. glottal
9. t _____		i. bilabial

2–7. Matching Phonetic Consonant Symbols to Manner Class

Match each individual or pair of phonetic symbols with the appropriate manner of articulation.

1. ʃ   _____
2. d͡ʒ   _____
3. l   _____
4. d   _____
5. w, ɹ _____
6. n   _____
7. w   _____

a. stop
b. nasal
c. glide
d. fricative
e. affricate
f. liquid
g. approximant

2–8. Matching Phonetic Consonant Symbols to Manner Class

Match each individual or pair of phonetic symbols to the appropriate manner of articulation.

1. j   _____
2. h   _____
3. t͡ʃ   _____
4. k   _____
5. ɹ   _____
6. m   _____

a. stop
b. nasal
c. glide
d. fricative
e. affricate
f. liquid

2–9. Describing Consonantal Articulation

Fill in the missing information.

Alphabetic Letter(s)	Phonetic Symbol	Voiced (+) or Voiceless (–)	Place of Articulation	Manner of Articulation
p				
d				
g				
n				
ng				
y				
v				
s				
sh				
h				
j				
r				

2–10. Describing Consonant Sounds in Words

Fill in the missing information for the bolded sound in each word.

Sound in Word	Phonetic Symbol	Word-Initial, Word-Medial, or Word-Final Position	Voiced (+) or Voiceless (–)	Place of Articulation	Manner of Articulation
bet					
bet					
catch					
catch					
woman					
woman					
bath					
bathe					
essay					
easy					
falling					
falling					

2–11. What Consonant Am I?

Determine the consonant phoneme(s) described by each clue.

1. I am a voiced bilabial glide.   _____

2. I am a voiceless alveolar stop.   _____

3. I am a voiceless post-alveolar fricative.   _____

4. I am a voiced velar stop.   _____

5. I am a voiceless glottal fricative.   _____

6. I am a voiced interdental fricative.   _____

7. I am a voiced retroflex liquid.   _____

8. I am a pair of alveolar fricatives.   _____

9. I am a voiced alveopalatal affricate.   _____

10. I am a voiced velar nasal.   _____

11. I am a voiced palatal glide.   _____

12. I am a voiceless bilabial stop.   _____

13. I am a voiceless alveolar fricative.   _____

14. I am a pair of labiodental fricatives.   _____

15. I am the cognate of /ð/.   _____

2–12. What Am I?

Read the clues to guess the word described.

1. I have a voiced alveolar stop in word-initial position.

   I turn into the crust of a pizza when baked.

   I am made of flour and tossed into the air.

   What am I?   _____

2. I have a voiced bilabial stop in word-medial position.

   I am a piece of furniture.

   I am surrounded by chairs.

   What am I?   _____

3. I have a voiceless velar stop in word-final position.

   I have words written inside of me.

   I can make you laugh or cry or even become smarter.

   What am I?   _____

4. I have a voiced bilabial nasal in word-initial position.

I am used to purchase things.

I am currency.

What am I?   _____

5. I have a voiced velar nasal in word-medial position.

I am used to keep clothes off the floor.

I am made of wood, plastic, or metal.

What am I?   _____

6. I have a voiced alveolar nasal in word-final position.

I am used to write on paper.

I have ink.

What am I?   _____

7. I have a voiced bilabial glide in word-medial position.

I look and smell nice.

I can be bought in a bouquet.

What am I?   _____

8. I have a voiced palatal glide in word-initial and word-medial positions.

I am a round toy you hold in your hand, and I have a long string to move me up and down.

Rock the baby, anyone?

What am I?   _____

9. I have a voiced labiodental fricative in word-initial position.

I am a decorative container.

I am made of glass, wood, or plastic.

What am I?   _____

10. I have a voiceless interdental fricative in word-initial position.

I am found on an extremity.

I am the opposable digit.

What am I? _____

11. I have a voiceless alveolar fricative in word-medial position.

I am a toddler eating spaghetti and meatballs with my fingers.

I am a child eating an ice cream cone on a hot summer day.

What am I? _____

12. I have a voiceless glottal fricative in word-medial position.

I am a popular internet search engine.

I also am an expression that usually is said with enthusiasm!

What am I? _____

13. I have a voiced alveopalatal affricate in word-initial position.

I am the place you go to work every day.

I am where you earn a living.

What am I? _____

14. I have a voiceless alveopalatal affricate in word-final position.

I am what you strike to make fire.

I come in a pack.

What am I? _____

15. I have a voiced palatal liquid in word-initial position.

I am the color of a Valentine's heart.

I am the color of blood.

What am I? _____

16. I have a voiced alveolar liquid in word-medial position.

I am a depth of water.

I am not deep.

What am I? _____

2–13. Building Words

Build words of the following phonotactic shapes using the designated consonants.

First, let's do one for practice: CVbV. Remember to focus on the sounds in words, not the orthographic letters.

What words might work for this pattern? Would *ruby*, *maybe*, *tube*, and *knobby* work?

The word *ruby* would work. It has four sounds: consonant sound [ɹ], long vowel sound "u," target consonant [b], and long vowel sound "e."

The word *maybe* would work too. It also has four sounds: consonant sound [m], long vowel sound "a," target sound [b], and long vowel sound "e."

The word *tube* would not work, even though it's spelled with four consonant-vowel-consonant-vowel letters, because the word *tube* has only three sounds: consonant sound [t], long vowel sound "u," and target sound [b]. The final letter "e" is silent.

Last, the word *knobby* would work. There are four sounds in *knobby*: consonant sound [n], vowel sound "ah," target consonant [b], and long vowel sound "e."

1. CVpV   _____

2. bVbV   _____

3. CVt   _____

4. dVd   _____

5. kCVC   _____

6. CVg   _____

7. CVmVC   _____

8. CVCVn   _____

9. CVŋVŋ   _____

10. wVC   _____

11. jVjV   _____

12. VfCVC   _____

13. VvVC   _____

14. CVθ   _____

15. CVð   _____

16. sCCVC   _____

17. CVz   _____

18. CVʃVC   _____

19. ʒVC   _____

20. VhV   _____

21. CVt͡ʃ   _____

22. d͡ʒVd͡ʒ   _____

23. CVlV   _____

24. ɹVCVC   _____

ARTICULATORY PHONETICS: VOWELS

3–1. Hearing Vowel Phonemes

Read the words for each question aloud. Listen carefully to the vowels. One word in each question has a different vowel phoneme. Circle the word with the differing vowel.

1.	book	should	hide	pull
2.	bead	sneak	said	cheese
3.	rid	fish	hitch	raw
4.	say	pail	trace	top
5.	aunt	kept	chest	bread
6.	cad	code	badge	bath
7.	couch	heart	marked	barn
8.	hood	cook	caught	push
9.	toe	snow	hot	ghost
10.	who	here	cruise	flew
11.	sir	snarl	search	curve
12.	man	tide	hive	sign
13.	how	loud	book	bough
14.	toy	boy	lone	coil
15.	sneer	tend	pier	beard
16.	dear	hair	chaired	prayer
17.	squire	tip	tires	higher
18.	cower	choir	sours	floured

3–2. Identifying Monophthong Vowel Phonemes in Orthographic Transcription

/i/

/i/ is the vowel in *bee, keen,* and *sea.* Circle which of the following words contain /i/.

soul	tree	pen	seize
heal	try	play	quit
dine	focus	queen	sigh
case	fly	cat	wash

/ɪ/

/ɪ/ is the vowel in *bit, kick,* and *chin.* Circle which of the following words contain /ɪ/.

speech	quite	mop	mint
heal	hymn	play	slit
dine	bear	loud	sigh
last	eel	squid	kit

/e/ - [eɪ]

[eɪ] is the frequent production of /e/ in *say, case,* and *late.* Circle which of the following words contain [eɪ].

feel	tree	vain	makes
heal	try	play	lamp
dine	bane	quail	chase
quake	phase	crab	blessed

/ɛ/

/ɛ/ is the vowel in *let, well,* and *gem.* Circle which of the following words contain /ɛ/.

case	tree	stench	choice
shell	mount	play	quit
knot	head	felt	traipse
now	goat	cat	beat

/æ/

/æ/ is the vowel in *bat, fast,* and *sack.* Circle which of the following words contain /æ/.

dough	baste	vain	trap
mop	spout	plaque	strength
ban	mouse	last	dozen
tree	case	thatch	say

/ʌ/

/ʌ/ is the vowel in *sun, just,* and *tuck.* Circle which of the following words contain /ʌ/.

bath	dug	end	fudge
goat	try	hurt	none
cut	bug	last	sigh
love	case	cough	strut

/ɝ/

/ɝ/ is the vowel in *shirt, burn,* and *her.* Circle which of the following words contain /ɝ/.

duck	fern	core	best
man	fire	church	swear
squirrel	twin	roar	surge
lark	fun	work	tired

/u/

/u/ is the vowel in *new, shoe,* and *pool.* Circle which of the following words contain /u/.

punt	blue	booth	mean
moon	brand	play	hall
strut	burn	choose	suit
who	fly	drew	book

/ʊ/

/ʊ/ is the vowel in *cook, would,* and *hood.* Circle which of the following words contain /ʊ/.

brood	budge	food	puts
rush	case	foot	squashed
dine	book	trend	pushed
could	try	first	last

/o/ - [o͡ʊ]

[o͡ʊ] is the typical production of /o/ in *low, go,* and *soak.* Circle which of the following words contain [o͡ʊ].

show	bond	goat	bone
hand	toast	spout	quit
broke	doubt	leaf	thought
mean	crowd	dough	posh

/ɔ/

/ɔ/ is the vowel in *log, saw,* and *thought.* Circle which of the following words contain /ɔ/. If you don't have /ɔ/ in your lexicon, circle the words that have /a/.

pool	put	dug	bought
whole	try	dough	hall
thaw	doze	trap	sigh
spout	case	envy	last

/ɑ/

/ɑ/ is the vowel in *hot, sock,* and *fall.* Circle which of the following words contain /ɑ/.

dine	enemy	watt	mean
cot	bad	play	quit
fly	mop	eel	case
knot	shot	trash	mom

3–3. Identifying Diphthong Vowel Phonemes in Orthographic Transcription

/aɪ/

/aɪ/ is the vowel in *fly, dime,* and *tie.* Circle which of the following words contain /aɪ/.

cried	vine	mean	psalm
heal	try	play	soup
dine	more	find	sigh
screech	case	skate	beat

/aʊ/

/aʊ/ is the vowel in *cow, shout,* and *ounce.* Circle which of the following words contain /aʊ/.

louse	now	friend	maze
feed	try	spout	mound
dine	books	splay	flipped
chair	crowd	glass	slouch

/ɔɪ/

/ɔɪ/ is the vowel in *boy, soil,* and *joy.* Circle which of the following words contain /ɔɪ/.

point	now	chips	mar
loud	choice	try	quit
dine	wolf	oil	toy
moist	shirt	cat	though

3–4. Identifying Rhotic Diphthongs and Triphthongs in Orthographic Transcription

/ɪɚ/

/ɪɚ/ is the vowel in *fear, cheered,* and *steers.* Circle which of the following words contain /ɪɚ/.

flirt	point	nor	fierce
clear	spheres	trees	quit
dine	bear	coin	year
wire	shirt	beard	cares

/ɛɚ/

/ɛɚ/ is the vowel in *bear, shared,* and *hair.* Circle which of the following words contain /ɛɚ/.

brash	cars	door	bared
tires	dare	rare	score
fair	brown	pliers	twist
moored	brawn	sure	blare

/ʊɚ/

/ʊɚ/ is the vowel in *cured* and *manure.* Circle which of the following words can contain /ʊɚ/. If this vowel phoneme is not in your lexicon, circle the words where you could produce [ʊɚ]

chord	tour	vent	bite
lure	bathe	cure	shard
toil	fjord	rear	chew

/ɔɚ/

/ɔɚ/ is the vowel in *boar, corn,* and *fort.* Circle which of the following words contain /ɔɚ/.

post	born	kale	pushed
glove	choice	worked	scorn
course	drive	look	plot
soar	worse	cat	quart

/ɑɚ/

/ɑɚ/ is the vowel in *barn, charge,* and *art.* Circle which of the following words contain /ɑɚ/.

swatch	spot	chai	farm
loud	chard	stork	spark
learn	boor	snarl	turn
coil	shirt	bush	bare

/aɪɚ/

/aɪɚ/ is the vowel in *ire, dryer,* and *briar.* Circle which of the following words contain /aɪɚ/.

cried	slow	board	parse
laud	thrice	dire	poor
dive	bear	oil	tire
hoist	higher	spire	roar

/aʊɚ/

/aʊɚ/ is the vowel in *our, showers,* and *powered.* Circle which of the following words contain /aʊɚ/.

cower	now	dirge	dour
loud	plaque	flour	lock
dine	bear	oil	tour
fire	shirt	tower	joke

3–5. Shared Vowel Phoneme

For each of the following questions, read the list of words aloud to yourself. You'll notice that one of the words in the list has a different vowel phoneme than the other words. Cross out the word that contains a different vowel. Add a word that shares the vowel phoneme of the remaining words.

1.	eight	that	shade	change	_____
2.	coat	down	hope	post	_____
3.	time	right	bite	make	_____
4.	lap	tap	neck	wag	_____
5.	cook	shoot	foot	hook	_____
6.	steep	check	neat	sheep	_____
7.	luck	hut	bug	chute	_____
8.	pig	bike	hip	trim	_____
9.	row	mouth	foul	vow	_____
10.	botch	joy	rot	shop	_____

3–6. Determining Type of Vowel

Tongue Advancement

Indicate whether each vowel is front, central, or back.

1. ʌ   front   central   back
2. e͡ɪ   front   central   back
3. ɪ   front   central   back
4. æ   front   central   back
5. ɛ   front   central   back
6. ɔ   front   central   back
7. ɚ   front   central   back
8. u   front   central   back
9. ʊ   front   central   back
10. i   front   central   back

Tongue Height

Indicate whether each vowel is high, mid, or low.

1. ɑ   high   mid   low
2. ʊ   high   mid   low
3. ʌ   high   mid   low
4. ɚ   high   mid   low
5. i   high   mid   low
6. ɛ   high   mid   low
7. æ   high   mid   low
8. u   high   mid   low
9. ɪ   high   mid   low
10. ɔ   high   mid   low

Lip Rounding

Indicate whether each vowel is rounded or unrounded.

1. ɑ   rounded   unrounded

2. ʊ   rounded   unrounded

3. ʌ   rounded   unrounded

4. ɝ   rounded   unrounded

5. i   rounded   unrounded

6. ɛ   rounded   unrounded

7. æ   rounded   unrounded

8. u   rounded   unrounded

9. ɪ   rounded   unrounded

10. ɔ   rounded   unrounded

3–7. Phonetic Transcription to English Orthographic Spelling

Read the following words. Write the English word that represents the phonemic transcription. There are three examples of each English vowel, including rhotic vowels.

1. a. /it/   _____
    b. /bif/   _____
    c. /wik/   _____

2. a. /kɑp/   _____
    b. /ʃɑk/   _____
    c. /sɑb/   _____

3. a. /fɪʃ/   _____
    b. /wɪt͡ʃ/   _____
    c. /θɪŋk/   _____

4. a. /d͡ʒɛt/   _____
    b. /ʃɛd/   _____
    c. /tɛst/   _____

5. a. /gæs/   _____

    b. /bæθ/   _____

    c. /ðæt/   _____

6. a. /stʌk/   _____

    b. /bʌnt͡ʃ/   _____

    c. /d͡ʒʌŋk/   _____

7. a. /d͡ʒɝm/   _____

    b. /ʃɝt/   _____

    c. /pɝt͡ʃ/   _____

8. a. /tuθ/   _____

    b. /t͡ʃuz/   _____

    c. /gus/   _____

9. a. /gʊd/   _____

    b. /kʊk/   _____

    c. /hʊd/   _____

10. a. /kɔt/   _____

    b. /ɹɔt/   _____

    c. /bɔt/   _____

11. a. /sket/   _____

    b. /wed͡ʒ/   _____

    c. /beʒ/   _____

12. a. /ɹot/   _____

    b. /ston/   _____

    c. /ðoz/   _____

13. a. /ka͡ɪt/   _____

    b. /ta͡ɪp/   _____

    c. /sa͡ɪn/   _____

14.   a.   /vɔɪd/   _____

      b.   /plɔɪ/   _____

      c.   /d͡ʒɔɪ/   _____

15.   a.   /sa͡ʊθ/   _____

      b.   /dɹa͡ʊt/   _____

      c.   /ka͡ʊt͡ʃ/   _____

16.   a.   /ji͡ɚz/   _____

      b.   /kli͡ɚ/   _____

      c.   /bi͡ɚd/   _____

17.   a.   /ʃɛ͡ɚ/   _____

      b.   /skwɛ͡ɚ/   _____

      c.   /t͡ʃɛ͡ɚz/   _____

18.   a.   /kju͡ɚ/   _____

      b.   /pju͡ɚ/   _____

      c.   /tu͡ɚd/   _____

19.   a.   /bɔ͡ɚd/   _____

      b.   /flɔ͡ɚ/   _____

      c.   /hɔ͡ɚs/   _____

20.   a.   /ʃɑ͡ɚp/   _____

      b.   /dɑ͡ɚk/   _____

      c.   /d͡ʒɑ͡ɚ/   _____

21.   a.   /ta͡ɪɚd/   _____

      b.   /wa͡ɪɚ/   _____

      c.   /pla͡ɪɚz/   _____

22.   a.   /a͡ʊɚ/   _____

      b.   /sa͡ʊɚ/   _____

      c.   /ska͡ʊɚd/   _____

3–8. Phonetic Transcription of Vowels

Practice writing the symbols for the vowels in the following words.

Sound	IPA Symbol	Transcription Practice
f<u>ee</u>t	i	
k<u>i</u>t	ɪ	
c<u>a</u>se	e͡ɪ	
br<u>ea</u>d	ɛ	
c<u>a</u>t	æ	
b<u>u</u>g	ʌ	
b<u>ir</u>d	ɝ	
f<u>oo</u>d	u	
t<u>oo</u>k	ʊ	
b<u>oa</u>t	o͡ʊ	
c<u>au</u>ght	ɔ	
h<u>o</u>t	ɑ	
s<u>igh</u>	a͡ɪ	
t<u>oy</u>	ɔ͡ɪ	
<u>ou</u>t	a͡ʊ	
f<u>ear</u>	i͡ɚ	
c<u>are</u>	ɛ͡ɚ	
t<u>our</u>	ʊ͡ɚ	
ch<u>ore</u>	ɔ͡ɚ	
t<u>ar</u>	ɑ͡ɚ	
h<u>ire</u>	a͡ɪɚ	
<u>our</u>	a͡ʊɚ	

3–9. Learning Vowel Descriptive Categories

Transcribe the following words using the International Phonetic Alphabet (IPA). You'll need to use the vowel symbols you have learned in Chapter 3 as well as the English consonant symbols you learned in Chapter 2.

Once you have transcribed the word, describe the vowel by each characteristic that applies. The first one has been done for you.

		Transcription	High, Mid, or Low?	Front, Central, or Back?	Lax or Tense?	Rounded or Unrounded?
1.	ask	æsk	low	front	lax	unrounded
2.	end					
3.	ill					
4.	geese					
5.	stew					
6.	shook					
7.	hug					
8.	soap					
9.	dock					
10.	bit					
11.	read					
12.	melt					
13.	pass					
14.	cruise					
15.	bush					
16.	bus					
17.	fox					
18.	deep					
19.	kick					

		Transcription	High, Mid, or Low?	Front, Central, or Back?	Lax or Tense?	Rounded or Unrounded?
20.	deck					
21.	perk					
22.	gum					
23.	face					
24.	book					
25.	knock					
26.	brook					
27.	run					
28.	lewd					
29.	elk					
30.	peel					

3–10. Shared Categories

Each of the following questions has three vowel phonemes listed. These three vowel phonemes share a common property. Please explain how the three vowels are alike.

1. /i/   /u/   /ʊ/   _____

2. /ɑ/   /u/   /i/   _____

3. /æ/   /ɪ/   /ɑ/   _____

4. /aɪ/   /ɪɚ/   /ɔɪ/   _____

5. /ʊ/   /ɝ/   /ɔ/   _____

6. /i/   /ɛ/   /e/   _____

7. /ɛ/   /ɔ/   /ʌ/   _____

8. /ɛ/   /ʊ/   /ɪ/   _____

9. /o/   /ʊ/   /ɑ/   _____

10. /aɪɚ/   /ɝ/   /ɪɚ/   _____

3–11. Discover the Vowel

Determine the vowel and the referenced word with the following information.

1. /b/ + high back vowel + /t/   Vowel: _____   Word: _____

2. /ɪ/ + mid central vowel + /f/   Vowel: _____   Word: _____

3. /p/ + low central diphthong +/t͡ʃ/   Vowel: _____   Word: _____

4. /b/ + low front vowel + /θ/   Vowel: _____   Word: _____

5. /ʃ/ + mid front vowel + /v/   Vowel: _____   Word: _____

6. /d͡ʒ/ + mid back vowel + /k/   Vowel: _____   Word: _____

7. /f/ + low back vowel + /l/   Vowel: _____   Word: _____

8. /t͡ʃ/ + mid front vowel + /k/   Vowel: _____   Word: _____

9. /d͡ʒ/ + mid back diphthong + /n/   Vowel: _____   Word: _____

10. /t/ + high front vowel + /p/   Vowel: _____   Word: _____

3–12. How Many Phonemes?

Count the phonemes in each of the following words. Hint: It will be easier to count phonemes if you transcribe each word before you get started.

1. frown   _____

2. brake   _____

3. jail   _____

4. scrunched   _____

5. wrath   _____

6. friend   _____

7. muse   _____

8. changed   _____

9. hope   _____

10. comb   _____

11. things _____

12. brook _____

13. feet _____

14. shorts _____

3–13. English Orthographic Spelling to Phonetic Transcription

Phonetically transcribe the following English words. The words are organized by vowel phoneme.

1. Words containing the high front tense unrounded vowel /i/.

   east _____   tree _____   neat _____   sheep _____   cheek _____

2. Words containing the high front lax unrounded vowel /ɪ/.

   tip _____   thick _____   lit _____   mist _____   fridge _____

3. Words containing the mid front to high front tense unrounded nonphonemic diphthong [eɪ].

   snake _____   they _____   cape _____   glaze _____   cage _____

4. Words containing the mid front lax unrounded vowel /ɛ/.

   stem _____   shed _____   jet _____   them _____   best _____

5. Words containing the low front lax unrounded vowel /æ/.

   batch _____   flap _____   track _____   badge _____   yak _____

6. Words containing the mid central lax unrounded vowel /ʌ/.

   truck _____   dutch _____   sunk _____   fudge _____   young _____

7. Words containing the mid central tense rounded vowel /ɝ/.

   perch _____   surge _____   first _____   third _____   yearn _____

8. Words containing the high back tense rounded vowel /u/.

   cute _____   boost _____   choose _____   fruit _____   coop _____

9. Words containing the high back lax rounded vowel /ʊ/.

   brook _____   could _____   crook _____   hook _____   stood _____

10. Words containing the mid back to high back rounded nonphonemic diphthong [o͡ʊ].

    joke _____   throat _____   ghost _____   show _____   vote _____

11. Words containing the mid back to high back rounded diphthong /ɔ/.

    caught _____   dog _____   flawed _____   taught _____   bought _____

12. Words containing the low back tense unrounded vowel /ɑ/.

    yacht _____   shock _____   botch _____   lox _____   squat _____

13. Words containing the low central to high front unrounded diphthong /a͡ɪ/.

    bite _____   slide _____   guy _____   white _____   type _____

14. Words containing the mid back rounded to high front unrounded diphthong /ɔ͡ɪ/.

    soil _____   joy _____   voice _____   coin _____   choice _____

15. Words containing the low central unrounded to high back rounded diphthong /a͡ʊ/.

    doubt _____   brown _____   cloud _____   shout _____   pouch _____

16. Words containing the rhotic diphthong /i͡ɚ/.

    jeer _____   dear _____   beers _____   smeared _____   cheer _____

17. Words containing the rhotic diphthong /ɛ͡ɚ/.

    blare _____   airs _____   chair _____   paired _____   square _____

18. Words containing the rhotic diphthong /ʊ͡ɚ/.

    lure _____   tour _____   pure _____   you're _____

19. Words containing the rhotic diphthong /ɔ͡ɚ/.

    quart _____   swarm _____   thwart _____   horse _____   court _____

20. Words containing the rhotic diphthong /a͡ɚ/.

    farm _____   jarred _____   hearth _____   charge _____   start _____

21. Words containing the rhotic triphthong /a͡ɪɚ/.

    pliers _____   mired _____   fire _____   friar _____   squire _____

22. Words containing the rhotic diphthong /a͡ʊɚ/.

    towers _____   showered _____   sour _____   power_____   our _____

3–14. Decipher the Vowel Phoneme

Fill in the blank with the appropriate vowel symbols from the description given. Then write the word in English orthography.

1. b___d   low, front   _____   _____

2. k___t   high, front   _____   _____

3. ʃ___t   high, back   _____   _____

4. k___p   mid, central   _____   _____

5. st___p   low, back   _____   _____

6. k___lt   mid, back   _____   _____

7. f___t   low, central   _____   _____

8. g___n   low, central   _____   _____

9. b___g   mid, front   _____   _____

10. t͡ʃ___f   high, front   _____   _____

3–15. Monophthong Versus Diphthong Versus Rhotic

For each of the following words, determine if the vowel <u>phoneme</u> is a monophthong, diphthong, or rhotic. After you have circled the correct choice, phonetically transcribe the word.

1. pit   monophthong   diphthong   rhotic   _____

2. bore   monophthong   diphthong   rhotic   _____

3. chat   monophthong   diphthong   rhotic   _____

4. shoot   monophthong   diphthong   rhotic   _____

5. owl   monophthong   diphthong   rhotic   _____

6. great   monophthong   diphthong   rhotic   _____

7. down   monophthong   diphthong   rhotic   _____

8. peer   monophthong   diphthong   rhotic   _____

9. shown   monophthong   diphthong   rhotic   _____

10. caught   monophthong   diphthong   rhotic   _____

11. teach   monophthong   diphthong   rhotic   _____

12. blurt   monophthong   diphthong   rhotic   _____

3–16. What Am I?

Read the clues and guess each word described. Write the word orthographically and phonetically.

1. My vowel is a monophthong or a nonphonemic diphthong.

   I am used to go from place to place quickly.

   I have pilots and flight attendants on my crew.

   What am I?   _____   _____

2. My vowel is a low, front monophthong.

   I am used in the game of baseball.

   I can be made from aluminum or wood.

   What am I?   _____   _____

3. My vowel is a phonemic diphthong.

   I will be an adult in my future.

   I like to play outside.

   What am I?   _____   _____

4. My vowel is a back diphthong.

   I have a painted face and a big red nose.

   I work in a circus.

   What am I?   _____   _____

5. My vowel is low and back.

   I am used to keep your feet warm.

   I only come in pairs.

   What am I?   _____   _____

6. My vowel is a phonemic diphthong.

   I have a tail and fly in the sky.

   I am traditionally the shape of a diamond.

   What am I?   _____   _____

7. My vowel is a high, back monophthong.

   I am used to hold your jackets or keys.

   I am the villain from Peter Pan.

   What am I?   _____   _____

8. My vowel is a rhotic monophthong.

   I begin and end with bilabial stops.

   I am a rude sound made while eating.

   What am I?   _____   _____

BROAD AND NARROW PHONETIC TRANSCRIPTION

4–1. Accurate or Inaccurate?

Determine whether each word that follows is transcribed accurately. Circle "yes "if accurate and "no" if the transcription is inaccurate. If the transcription is incorrect, transcribe the word correctly on the line provided. Note that errors can be consonant or vowel phonemes.

1. knit   /nɪt/   Accurate: Yes / No   _____

2. tough   /tɑf/   Accurate: Yes / No   _____

3. quest   /qwɛst/   Accurate: Yes / No   _____

4. bush   /bʊʃ/   Accurate: Yes / No   _____

5. sung   /sɑŋ/   Accurate: Yes / No   _____

6. bath   /bæθ/   Accurate: Yes / No   _____

7. switch   /swɪt͡ʃ/   Accurate: Yes / No   _____

8. worm   /wɔ͡ɚm/   Accurate: Yes / No   _____

9. guard   /gɑ͡ɚd/   Accurate: Yes / No   _____

10. wrote   /wɹo͡ʊt/   Accurate: Yes / No   _____

4–2. Phonetic Transcription: Stops, Nasals, and Glides With Front Vowels

Phonetically transcribe each word after identifying the number of phonemes in each word.

Word	# of Phonemes	Phonetic Transcription
win		
bean		
man		
at		
pant		
dig		
kin		
bend		
yam		
meat		
beat		
beg		
bent		
king		
mend		

4–3. Phonetic Transcription: Stops, Nasals, and Glides With Front Vowels

Phonetically transcribe each word after identifying the number of phonemes in each word.

Word	# of Phonemes	Phonetic Transcription
pat		
bed		
pet		
knee		
bin		
mint		
quit		
nag		
bet		
be		
key		
camp		
mat		
yet		
bang		

4–4. Phonetic Transcription: Stops, Nasals, and Glides With Central and Back Vowels

Phonetically transcribe each word after identifying the number of phonemes in each word.

Word	# of Phonemes	Phonetic Transcription
nut		
boot		
dog		
book		
wand		
took		
cough		
suit		
not		
want		
tug		
dot		
tong		
cut		
you		

4–5. Phonetic Transcription: Stops, Nasals, and Glides With Central and Back Vowels

Phonetically transcribe each word after identifying the number of phonemes in each word.

Word	# of Phonemes	Phonetic Transcription
yawn		
taught		
what		
pun		
bump		
gone		
nook		
mood		
daunt		
boo		
young		
lot		
wood		
on		
doom		

4–6. Phonetic Transcription: Stops, Nasals, and Glides With Diphthong Vowels

Phonetically transcribe each word after identifying the number of phonemes in each word.

Word	# of Phonemes	Phonetic Transcription
mine		
wait		
boy		
cow		
boat		
toe		
pain		
buy		
gaze		
time		
mount		
coin		
goat		
point		
town		

4–7. Phonetic Transcription: Stops, Nasals, and Glides With Diphthong Vowels

Phonetically transcribe each word after identifying the number of phonemes in each word.

Word	# of Phonemes	Phonetic Transcription
toy		
now		
toad		
cake		
white		
might		
dime		
out		
oink		
dome		
comb		
boink		
bang		
whine		
count		

4–8. Phonetic Transcription: Stops, Nasals, and Glides With Rhotic Vowels

Phonetically transcribe each word after identifying the number of phonemes in each word.

Word	# of Phonemes	Phonetic Transcription
bird		
year		
bear		
our		
core		
arm		
tour		
earn		
yarn		
tire		
gear		
cure		
war		
dire		
more		

4–9. Phonetic Transcription: Stops, Nasals, and Glides With Rhotic Vowels

Phonetically transcribe each word after identifying the number of phonemes in each word.

Word	# of Phonemes	Phonetic Transcription
term		
deer		
pure		
court		
yard		
carp		
dirt		
pear		
park		
wire		
board		
card		
hour		
born		
wear		

4–10. Phonetic Transcription: Fricatives, Affricates, and Liquids With Front Vowels

Phonetically transcribe each word after identifying the number of phonemes in each word.

Word	# of Phonemes	Phonetic Transcription
cheese		
fish		
sledge		
sash		
seal		
gel		
rash		
have		
thief		
sill		
ledge		
this		
etch		
she		
wrath		

4–11. Phonetic Transcription: Fricatives, Affricates, and Liquids With Front Vowels

Phonetically transcribe each word after identifying the number of phonemes in each word.

Word	# of Phonemes	Phonetic Transcription
flash		
is		
chief		
freeze		
hedge		
with		
less		
jazz		
flesh		
these		
veal		
stitch		
says		
seize		
hatch		

4–12. Phonetic Transcription: Fricatives, Affricates, and Liquids With Central and Back Vowels

Phonetically transcribe each word after identifying the number of phonemes in each word.

Word	# of Phonemes	Phonetic Transcription
judge		
love		
shawl		
the		
full		
shoes		
hot		
huge		
chew		
jaw		
fall		
lock		
saw		
sludge		
rule		

4–13. Phonetic Transcription: Fricatives, Affricates, and Liquids With Central and Back Vowels

Phonetically transcribe each word after identifying the number of phonemes in each word.

Word	# of Phonemes	Phonetic Transcription
soothe		
shook		
fuzz		
through		
shove		
choose		
push		
raw		
use		
rush		
shot		
hall		
zoo		
juice		
loss		

4–14. Phonetic Transcription: Fricatives, Affricates, and Liquids With Diphthong Vowels

Phonetically transcribe each word after identifying the number of phonemes in each word.

Word	# of Phonemes	Phonetic Transcription
save		
loaf		
south		
life		
soy		
change		
rice		
oil		
those		
chow		
soul		
choice		
file		
sale		
vow		

4–15. Phonetic Transcription: Fricatives, Affricates, and Liquids With Diphthong Vowels

Phonetically transcribe each word after identifying the number of phonemes in each word.

Word	# of Phonemes	Phonetic Transcription
joust		
lie		
soil		
chase		
hose		
voice		
jail		
sigh		
though		
mouth		
how		
joy		
raise		
slow		
five		

4–16. Phonetic Transcription: Fricatives, Affricates, and Liquids With Rhotic Vowels

Phonetically transcribe each word after identifying the number of phonemes in each word.

Word	# of Phonemes	Phonetic Transcription
lure		
fair		
verse		
shore		
tsar		
surf		
there		
veer		
sour		
hair		
fear		
church		
roar		
higher		
sheer		

4–17. Phonetic Transcription: Fricatives, Affricates, and Liquids With Rhotic Vowels

Phonetically transcribe each word after identifying the number of phonemes in each word.

Word	# of Phonemes	Phonetic Transcription
earth		
sewer		
flour		
jar		
cheer		
sore		
liar		
share		
chore		
chairs		
fire		
shower		
fur		
here		
far		

4–18. Phonetic Transcription: Disyllabic Words With Front Vowels

Phonetically transcribe each word after identifying the number of phonemes in each word.

Word	# of Phonemes	Phonetic Transcription
vaccine		
taxes		
eggshell		
palate		
heaven		
receipt		
basket		
sibling		
discrete		
lefty		
petite		
festive		
prison		
treason		
fencing		

4–19. Phonetic Transcription: Disyllabic Words With Front Vowels

Phonetically transcribe each word after identifying the number of phonemes in each word.

Word	# of Phonemes	Phonetic Transcription
sheepish		
kitten		
magnet		
caption		
teaches		
decrease		
acting		
trapeze		
lesson		
wagon		
helmet		
lettuce		
gallop		
napkin		
zigzag		

4–20. Phonetic Transcription: Disyllabic Words With Central and Back Vowels

Phonetically transcribe each word after identifying the number of phonemes in each word.

Word	# of Phonemes	Phonetic Transcription
jumpy		
crouton		
rebuke		
spoonful		
juggle		
trouble		
cocoon		
also		
awful		
costume		
bubble		
hubris		
stubble		
muscle		
unhook		

4–21. Phonetic Transcription: Disyllabic Words With Central and Back Vowels

Phonetically transcribe each word after identifying the number of phonemes in each word.

Word	# of Phonemes	Phonetic Transcription
fungus		
chocolate		
balloon		
quota		
jungle		
glucose		
bottle		
oblong		
pupil		
cuckoo		
judo		
bugle		
mushroom		
couple		
pontoon		

4–22. Phonetic Transcription: Disyllabic Words With All Vowels

Phonetically transcribe each word after identifying the number of phonemes in each word.

Word	# of Phonemes	Phonetic Transcription
locket		
outdo		
baboon		
downy		
renowned		
eyelash		
input		
storage		
convoy		
dormant		
ozone		
chicken		
deter		
repair		
reading		

4–23. Phonetic Transcription: Disyllabic Words With All Vowels

Phonetically transcribe each word after identifying the number of phonemes in each word.

Word	# of Phonemes	Phonetic Transcription
chipmunk		
safety		
message		
journey		
mermaid		
tackle		
thoughtful		
disease		
issue		
shovel		
pulley		
outlook		
causeway		
tarmac		
exploit		

4–24. Phonetic Transcription: Polysyllabic Words With All Vowels

Phonetically transcribe each word after identifying the number of phonemes in each word.

Word	# of Phonemes	Phonetic Transcription
recycle		
firemen		
ponytail		
triangle		
application		
advantage		
amplifier		
knowingly		
judgment		
enlighten		
holiday		
beginning		
tableware		
unicorn		
piggy bank		

4–25. Phonetic Transcription: Polysyllabic Words With All Vowels

Phonetically transcribe each word after identifying the number of phonemes in each word.

Word	# of Phonemes	Phonetic Transcription
rectangle		
president		
language		
ordinary		
exchange		
disqualify		
confidence		
thousand		
minority		
buoyant		
zucchini		
everything		
quintuplet		
Blackbeard		
themselves		

4–26. Phonetic Transcription: Polysyllabic Words With All Vowels

Phonetically transcribe each word after identifying the number of phonemes in each word.

Word	# of Phonemes	Phonetic Transcription
childhood		
bullying		
coordinate		
annual		
relaxation		
invisible		
adversity		
forgiveness		
insomniac		
captivate		
ignition		
jellyfish		
obesity		
Thursday		
exhaling		

4–27. Phonetic Transcription: Same-Vowel Phrases

Phonetically transcribe each phrase.

Phrase	Phonetic Transcription
flea sneezed	
shrimp primped	
whale ailed	
hen bent	
cat sat	
bug hugged	
bird heard	
moose mused	
wolf put	
roach joked	
hog brawled	
fox trotted	
fly sighed	
chow-chow bowed	
koi destroyed	

4–28. Reading Phonetic Transcription: Same-Vowel Phrases

Orthographically write each phonetically transcribed phrase. Remember that there are no capital phonetic symbols.

Phonetic Transcription	Phrase
[li bimz]	
[d͡ʒɪl bɪldz]	
[d͡ʒeɪd eɪks]	
[bɛl bɛts]	
[æn ækts]	
[t͡ʃʌk wʌn]	
[pɚl wɝlz]	
[kɹuz t͡ʃuz]	
['wʊ.di lʊks]	
[bo͡ʊ d͡ʒo͡ʊks]	
[pɑl nɑz] - [pɔl nɔz]	
[tɑʒ dɹɑps]	
[ma͡ɪ kɹa͡ɪz]	
[kla͡ʊs ha͡ʊlz]	
[ɹɔ͡ɪ d͡ʒɔ͡ɪnz]	

4–29. Reading Phonetic Transcription: Front Vowels With Different Spellings

Orthographically write each phonetically transcribed word.

Phonetic Transcription	Word
[ni]	
[ki]	
[mi]	
[si]	
[snɪf]	
['wɪ.mɪn] - ['wɪ.mən]	
[θɹɛd]	
[sɛd]	
[bɛd]	
[kætʃ]	
[kæn]	

4–30. Reading Phonetic Transcription: Central and Back Vowels With Different Spellings

Orthographically write each phonetically transcribed word.

Phonetic Transcription	Word
[lʌʃ]	
[dʌn]	
[blɑg] - [blɔg]	
[hɑt] - [hɔt]	
[mun]	
[tun]	
[hʊd]	
[ʃʊd]	
[ɑt] - [ɔt]	
[kɑt] - [kɔt]	

4–31. Reading Phonetic Transcription: Diphthongs With Different Spellings

Orthographically write each phonetically transcribed word.

Phonetic Transcription	Word
[taɪ]	
[saɪ]	
[flaɪ]	
[haɪ]	
[haɪst̚]	
[baɪt]	
[baʊ.waʊ]	
[plaʊd]	
[bɔɪz]	
[nɔɪz]	
[ɹeɪ]	
[weɪ]	
[weɪst]	
[weɪt]	
[koʊm]	
[hoʊm]	

4–32. Diacritical Marks for Consonants

1. Match each state of the glottis with its corresponding diacritical mark.

   voiceless _____   a. [x̪]

   aspirated _____   b. [xʰ]

   voiced _____   c. [x̥]

   creaky _____   d. [x̰]

2. Narrowly transcribe each of the following words using the appropriate diacritical mark.

   a. *teeth* produced with tongue tip touching the back of the upper   _____
   incisors for /t/

   b. *zoo* produced with blade of the tongue used to produce [z]   _____

   c. *one* produced with a nasalized word-initial consonant   _____

   d. *zip* produced by lateralizing [z]   _____

   e. *tap* produced by unreleasing the word-final stop phoneme   _____

   f. *juice* produced by prolonging the final consonant   _____

   g. *bottle* produced with a syllabic final consonant   _____

4–33. Marking Primary Stress in Disyllabic Words

Include the primary stress diacritic in your phonetic transcription of each of the following prepositions.

1. beside   _____

2. anti   _____

3. during   _____

4. within   _____

5. versus   _____

6. into   _____

7. beyond   _____

8. inside   _____

9. onto   _____

10. without   _____

4–34. Using the Tap Allophone

Circle "yes" or "no" to indicate whether the /t/ or /d/ phoneme can be replaced by a tap. Then phonetically transcribe each word, using the tap allophone where possible. If the tap cannot be used, briefly explain why.

1. letter   yes / no   _____   If no: No, because _____ .

2. watt   yes / no   _____   If no: No, because _____ .

3. cattail   yes / no   _____   If no: No, because _____ .

4. cigarette   yes / no   _____   If no: No, because _____ .

5. little   yes / no   _____   If no: No, because _____ .

6. ditto   yes / no   _____   If no: No, because _____ .

7. attack   yes / no   _____   If no: No, because _____ .

8. attic   yes / no   _____   If no: No, because _____ .

9. attention   yes / no   _____   If no: No, because _____ .

10. odd   yes / no   _____   If no: No, because _____ .

11. adding   yes / no   _____   If no: No, because _____ .

12. addition   yes / no   _____   If no: No, because _____ .

13. cheddar   yes / no   _____   If no: No, because _____ .

14. buddy   yes / no   _____   If no: No, because _____ .

15. ado   yes / no   _____   If no: No, because _____ .

5

SUPRASEGMENTAL FEATURES OF SPEECH

5–1. Stress: Identifying and Diagramming Stress in Words

Underline the stressed syllables in each pair of words. Then diagram the stress pattern. An example has been done for you.

Example:

    instant   inform

    ————   ————

        ————   ————

    __in__   stant   in   __form__

1. unless   under

2. effect   affect

3. supper   support

4. between   beacon

5. beckon   because

6. about   able

7. away   awesome

8. disagree   disaggregate

9. against   agency

10. acre   across

11. agate   again

12. around   Arabic

13. between   Beatrice

14. Beckman   because

15. canopy   control

16. create   crease

17. himself   hymnal

18. pumice   police

19. until   unanimous

20. wither   within

21. witness   without

22. polar   polite

5–2. Stress: Identifying Stress in Different Forms of the Same Word

Underline the stressed syllables in the following words.

1. interpret   interpreter   interpretation

2. wonder   wonderful   wonderfully

3. remain   remainder   remaining

4. icon   iconic   iconicity

5. agree   agreement   agreeable

6. apply   applicant   application

7. advertise   advertising   advertisement

8. believe   believable   believability

9. ideal   idealize   ideally

10. navigate   navigator   navigation

11. lemon   lemonade

12. king   kingdom

5–3. Syntactic Phrases: Saying One Utterance Using Two Different Phrase Units

Produce each utterance using two different phrase units.

1. Let's cook grandpa dinner tonight.

   _____

   _____

2. I saw a man eating chicken.

   _____

   _____

3. Twenty five dollar bills.

_____

_____

4. It's raining children.

_____

_____

5. I'm sorry I love you.

_____

_____

6. I find joy in cooking my family and my dog.

_____

_____

5–4. Intonation: Saying Sentences With Specified Intonation Contours

Practice saying each utterance using the intonation contour diagrammed.

1. I saw you yesterday.

2. I saw you yesterday?

3. She likes burgers and fries.

        ―――

          ―――

―――   ―――   ―――

―――

4. Did your brother text you?

        ―――

      ―――

    ―――

―――   ―――   ―――

5. What time will you be ready?

  ―――

    ―――

―――   ―――   ―――   ―――＼

5–5. Intonation: Saying Sentences With Specified Intonation Contours

Write an utterance that could fit each intonation contour diagrammed.

1. _____

  ―――

――― ――― ―――

    ―――＼

2. _____

    ―――／

    ――― ―――

――― ―――

3. _____

4. _____

5. _____

5–6. Prosody: Saying One Utterance Using Two Different Phrase Units

Practice saying each of the following nonsense phrases until you come up with a commonly used term.

1. foe net ick sigh ants   _____

2. overt a reign bow   _____

3. are tick you lay shun   _____

4. poor to Lynn door a gun   _____

5. bolt Tim more merry Lynn   _____

6. cam bow Dee ha   _____

7. wall diss knee   _____

8. hair reap otter   _____

9. jewel yeehaw rob hurts   _____

10. chess ape eek bay _____

11. wheel ute ants we the me _____

12. kid tea vee dee oh _____

ACOUSTIC PHONETICS

6–1. Acoustic Terms

1. A wave resulting from an up and down movement wave that travels side to side is a
    _____ wave.

2. If a movement and the resulting pressure wave travel in the same direction the wave is
    _____.

3. Sound waves are which type of wave? _____

4. When molecules are farther apart from each than they are in their resting position, it is
    called _____.

5. Molecules that are closer together than they are in their resting position are in a state
    called _____.

6. Air pressure variations over time can be graphed on a _____.

7. Decibels measure intensity / frequency. (Choose one)

8. Hertz measure intensity / frequency. (Choose one)

6–2. Acoustic Phonetic Terms

1. Frequency is the objective representation of _____.

2. Loudness is a subjective representation of _____.

3. How are frequency and time related?

    _____

    _____

    _____

4. Define fundamental frequency.

_____

_____

_____

5. What fundamental frequency differences are observed between biological males and biological females? What differences in fundamental frequency are observed between adults and children?

_____

_____

_____

6–3. Waveforms

1. Is the following waveform periodic or aperiodic? How can you tell?

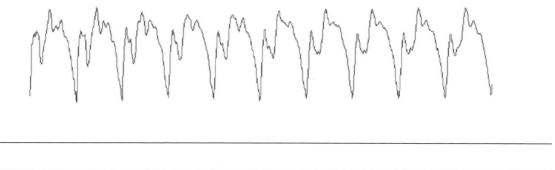

_____

_____

2. Which of the following waveforms shows a pure tone? Which of the following shows speech?

A.

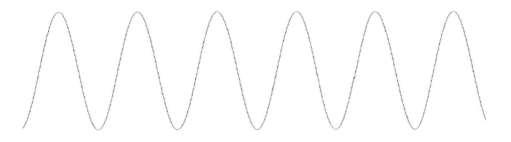

B.

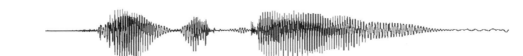

6–4. Calculating Fundamental Frequency

1. The duration of the following Waveform A is 0.044 s. Calculate F0:

Waveform A

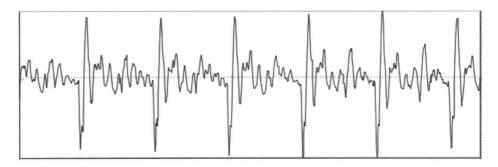

2. The duration of the following Waveform B is .029 s. Calculate F0:

Waveform B

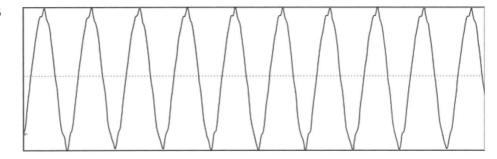

3. The duration of the following Waveform C is .038 s. Calculate F0:

Waveform C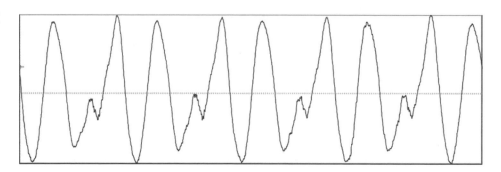

_____

4. Which of the previous waveforms has the highest F0? The lowest F0?

_____

_____

_____

6–5. Waveform Word Matching

1. Match the waveforms to the five words that follow. How did you make each decision?

stop   beep   four   aim   witch

A.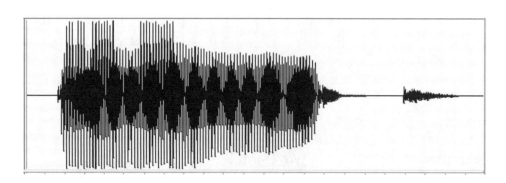

Waveform A is of the word _____

_____

_____

B.

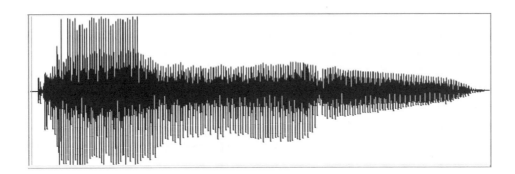

Waveform B is of the word _____

_____

_____

C.

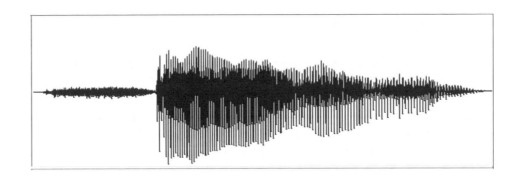

Waveform C is of the word _____

_____

_____

D.

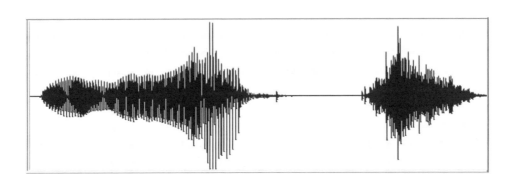

Waveform D is of the word _____

_____

_____

E.

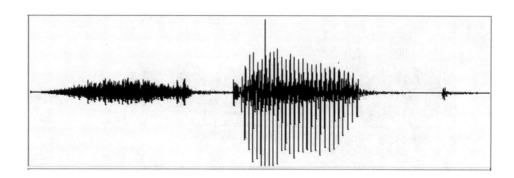

Waveform E is of the word _____

_____

_____

6–6. Spectrogram Definitions

1. On a spectrogram, what is the relationship between F1 and tongue height? F2 and tongue advancement?

_____

_____

2. For the following vowels, describe the expected F1 and F2 based on tongue placement.

[u]: _____

_____

[i]: _____

_____

[æ]: _____

_____

[ɑ]: _____

_____

[aɪ]: _____

_____

6–7. Articulatory Versus Acoustic Space for Vowels

1. On the following grid, plot the vowels in the acoustic space. Each tick mark on the grid is 100 Hz.

   Vowel 1. F1: 280 F2: 2300

   Vowel 2. F1: 700 F2: 2000

   Vowel 3. F1: 640 F2: 1250

   Vowel 4. F1: 320 F2: 1300

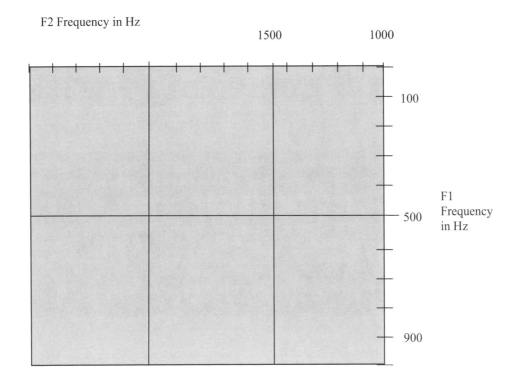

2. Identify these four vowel phonemes based on their position in the acoustic space.

   a. Vowel 1: _____

   b. Vowel 2: _____

   c. Vowel 3: _____

   d. Vowel 4: _____

6–8. Spectrogram Vowel Matching

Match the following spectrograms with the monophthong or diphthong vowels. Explain the acoustic features that were used to match the vowel to the spectrogram.

[ɔɪ]   [ɪ]   [ɑ]   [aʊ]   [u]

A.

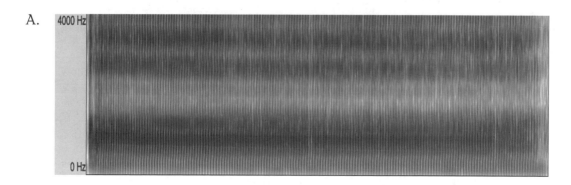

B.

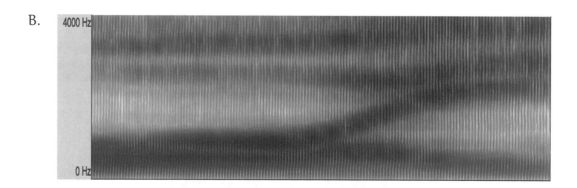

C.

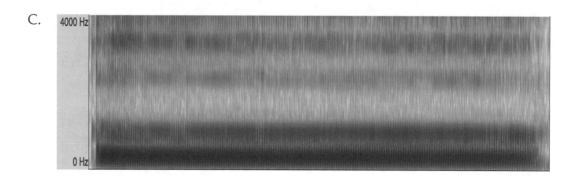

D.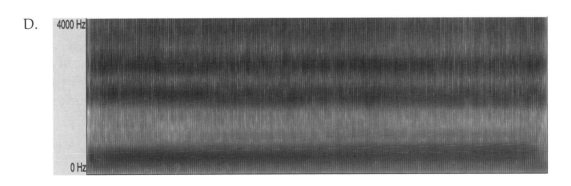

E.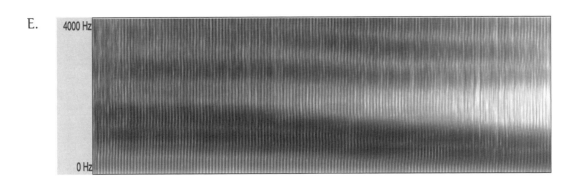

a. _____

_____

_____

b. _____

_____

_____

c. _____

_____

_____

d. _____

_____

_____

e. _____

_____

_____

6–9. Matching Spectrograms

Spectrograms A through F are of [ʌ.Cʌ] productions, the [C] representing a consonant phoneme of English. Each spectrogram shows acoustic energy from 0 to 4000 Hz. Match the following consonant phonemes to their spectrogram, briefly describing how you found your answer.

[m]   [k]   [s]   [d͡ʒ]   [ʃ]   [ɹ]

A.

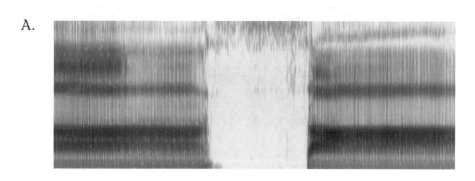

B.

C.

D.

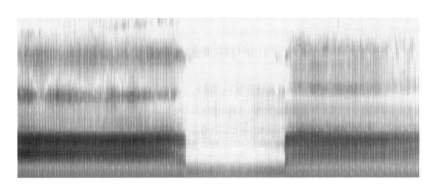

E.

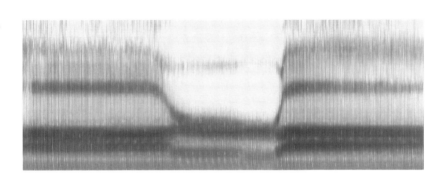

F.

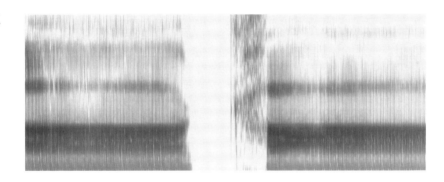

Spectrogram A: _____

_____

_____

_____

Spectrogram B: _____

_____

_____

_____

Spectrogram C: _____

_____

_____

_____

Spectrogram D: _____

_____

_____

_____

Spectrogram E: _____

_____

_____

_____

Spectrogram F: _____

_____

_____

_____

6–10. Segmenting Waveforms

The following six words are represented in the following spectrograms—spectrogram A, B, and C. There are two words in each spectrogram. Match each word to its corresponding spectrogram. Below each spectrogram, transcribe each word and segment each spectrogram.

doom   *ballistic*   *statistic*   *mines*   *mood*   *prince*

A.

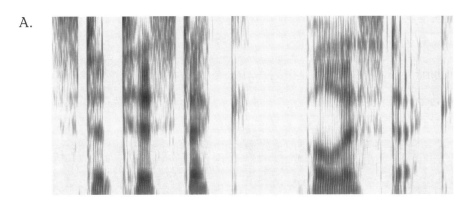

B.

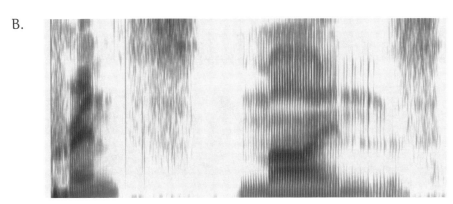

C.

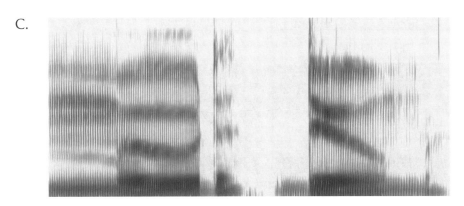

Spectrogram A: _____

Spectrogram B: _____

Spectrogram C: _____

6–11. Spectrogram Sentence Reading

Match each of the following spectrograms—labeled A, B, and C—with one of the following phrases. There are extra phrases provided to increase the challenge.

Run really fast.

It's time.

The dog is outside.

Hang on to my ring.

Please stop and think.

What is the answer to the question?

A.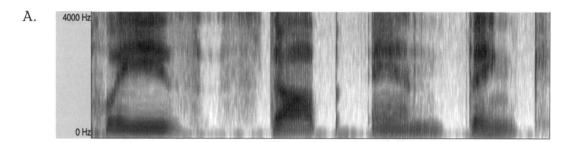

B.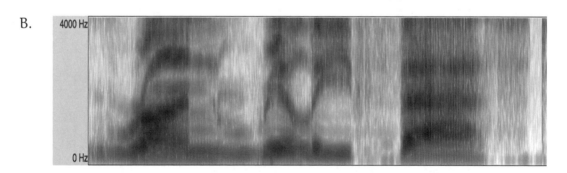

C.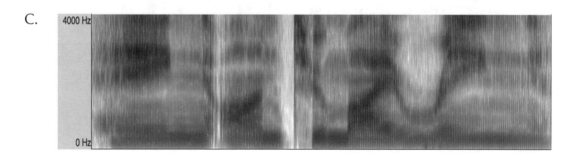

Spectrogram A: _____

Spectrogram B: _____

Spectrogram C: _____

6–12. Try It Yourself: Wavesurfer and Praat Download Links

Try making your own waveforms and spectrograms with the free downloadable software, Wavesurfer or Praat! You can explore different user interfaces and capabilities using these software.

Free Praat download for Windows:
http://www.fon.hum.uva.nl/praat/download_win.html

Free Praat download for Mac:
http://www.fon.hum.uva.nl/praat/download_mac.html

Free Wavesurfer download at https://sourceforge.net/projects/wavesurfer/

7

CONSONANT PHONOLOGY

7–1. Syllabicity: Identifying Parts of Syllables

Fill in the missing information.

Orthographic Transcription	Phonetic Transcription	Onset	Rime	Nucleus	Coda
send					
tries					
mist					
act					
bee					
play					
crooks					
lunch					

7–2. Stops: Identifying Words With Syllable-Initial Aspiration

Circle the words for which the syllable-initial stop aspiration rule could apply.

taxi	stay	carrot	baggage
paper	letter	apple	cook
baton	native	king	speak
kick	winner	two	novice
money	target	park	slate
upon	music	skill	economy
rain	witch	fake	support

7–3. Stops: Identifying and Transcribing Words With Syllable-Initial Aspiration

Circle the word in each pair for which the syllable-initial stop aspiration rule could apply. Then transcribe each word.

Word A	Word B	Transcription A	Transcription B
squid	kid	_____	_____
atop	stop	_____	_____
bobbing	popping	_____	_____
stark	tarp	_____	_____
toggle	boggle	_____	_____
carry	scary	_____	_____
spot	pot	_____	_____
bye	pie	_____	_____

7–4. Stops: Identifying Words With Word-Final Unreleased Stops

Circle the words for which the word-final unreleased stop rule could apply.

ship	back	dome	top
fire	mat	doctor	chalet
rot	cheese	pick	loss
lamb	farm	can't	salt
rope	patch	myth	map
complete	swirl	buzz	attack

7–5. Stops: Identifying and Transcribing Words With Word-Final Unreleased Stops

Circle the word in each pair for which the word-final unreleased stop rule could apply. Then transcribe each word.

Word A	Word B	Transcription A	Transcription B
can't	band		
shrug	shuck		
hip	glib		
grand	art		
teacup	bathtub		
walled	wallet		
bullfrog	garlic		
plate	played		
loop	lobe		
bag	back		
knit	node		
snip	crib		

7–6. Stops: Identifying Words With Unreleased Stops in Stop + Stop Clusters or When Preceding Syllabic Nasals

1. Circle the words for which the unreleased stop in a stop + stop cluster rule could apply.

wagged	whipped	trucked	dictate
inducted	baked	haste	hoped
bacteria	octopus	bracelet	fiction
teacher	doctor	lawyer	engineer

2. Circle the words for which the unreleased stop preceding a syllabic nasal rule could apply.

kitten	fasten	fashion	lighten
atom	fatten	satin	settle
mission	kitchen	leaden	batten
sadden	bottom	lentil	even

7–7. Stops: Identifying Words With Unaspirated Stops in /s/ + Stop Clusters

Circle the words for which the unaspirated stop in /s/ + stop cluster rule could apply.

scene	spill	sky	stop
style	scam	psychology	mister
fasten	skip	scale	speckle
slap	scent	spam	scythe
whisker	swan	school	square
rescue	chopstick	sweater	spatula
haystack	snowstorm	teaspoon	basket

7–8. Stops: Identifying and Transcribing Words With Unaspirated Stops in /s/ + Stop Clusters

Circle the word in each pair for which the unaspirated stop in /s/ + stop clusters rule could apply. Then transcribe each word.

Word A	Word B	Transcription A	Transcription B
scale	kale		
sunk	skunk		
slid	skid		
smile	style		
smoke	spoke		
costume	consume		
telescope	telephone		
snow	storm		
banister	banish		
sting	swing		
busy bee	biscuit		
apostrophe	apology		

7–9. Stops: Identifying and Transcribing Words With Labialized Stops

Circle the words for which the labialized rule could apply to the stop preceding the vowel. Then transcribe each word.

Word	Transcription
poke	_____
beat	_____
took	_____
dime	_____
quick	_____
goose	_____
pop	_____
boot	_____
take	_____
dome	_____
squirt	_____
good	_____

7–10. Stops: Identifying and Transcribing Words With Dentalized Alveolar Stops

Circle the words for which the dentalized rule could apply to the alveolar stop preceding /θ/. Then transcribe each word.

Word	Transcription
length	_____
width	_____
breadth	_____
depth	_____
bandwidth	_____
hundredth	_____
birthday	_____
mythical	_____
thousandth	_____
eighth	_____

7–11. Stops: Identifying and Transcribing Words With Advanced Velar Stops

Circle the words for which the advanced velar stop rule could apply. Then transcribe each word.

Word	Transcription
keep	_____
kept	_____
cop	_____
cape	_____
ghost	_____
give	_____
get	_____
goose	_____
weak	_____
woke	_____
stick	_____
sag	_____

7–12. Stops: Identifying and Transcribing Words With Glottal Replacements

Circle the word in each pair for which the alveolar stop preceding a syllabic /n/ is replaced with a glottal stop rule could apply. Then transcribe each word.

Word A	Word B	Transcription A	Transcription B
kitten	bottom		
leaden	sweater		
written	tomato		
doctor	fightin'		
Sweden	sweeter		
baton	rotten		
sagging	satin		
heighten	butter		
battery	button		

7–13. Stops: Identifying and Transcribing Words With Nasal Releases

Circle the words for which the stop preceding a syllabic nasal is released with nasal plosion rule could apply. Then transcribe each word.

Word   Transcription

sadden   _____

shouldn't   _____

vacuum   _____

happen   _____

become   _____

couldn't   _____

ignite   _____

upon   _____

burden   _____

administer   _____

succumb   _____

mannequin   _____

7–14. Stops: Transcribing Words With Lateral Releases

Circle the correct transcription for each of the following words for which the lateral release in stop + /l/-clusters rule can apply.

cloud	kɫaʊ͡d	kˡla͡ʊd	cla͡ʊd
plate	pʰle͡ɪt	pɫe͡ɪt	pˡle͡ɪt
clue	kˡlue	kˡlu	kɫu
blow	bˡlo͡ʊ	blo	bɫo͡ʊ
blade	bˡle͡ɪd	bɫe͡ɪd	bˡlade
glass	gɫæs	gˡlæss	gˡlæs
climb	kɫim	kˡla͡ɪmb	kˡla͡ɪm
glue	gˡɫu	gɫu	gˡlu
black	bˡlæk	bˡlæck	bɫæk
glove	gɫʌv	gˡlʌv	gɫvʌ
clock	kˡlæk	kɫæk	kˡlɑk
pluck	pɫuk	pˡɫʌk	pˡlʌk

7–15. Stops: Transcribing Words With Affricated Alveolar Stops

Use narrow transcription to transcribe the following words, demonstrating allophonic affrication.

Word	Transcription
tree	_____
dress	_____
try	_____
dry	_____
tray	_____
drink	_____
truck	_____
drove	_____
metric	_____
address	_____

7–16. Stops: Transcribing Words With Word-Medial Taps

Pay attention to whether the medial stop is pronounced as /t/, /d/, or /ɾ/. Circle the words containing a tap phone. Then transcribe each word.

Word	Transcription
butter	_____
middle	_____
pretty	_____
valentine	_____
ladder	_____
drumstick	_____

Word	Transcription
vitamin	_____
addendum	_____
military	_____
pity	_____
matter	_____
hotel	_____
water	_____
addition	_____
mighty	_____
putter	_____
noodle	_____
cactus	_____
stutter	_____
litter	_____
sledding	_____
bathtub	_____
kitty	_____
address	_____
lunchtime	_____
flighty	_____
photo	_____
spotty	_____

7–17. Stops: Identifying and Transcribing Utterances With Stop Shortening

Say each utterance aloud, paying attention to whether both stops in doubled contexts are fully articulated. Circle the word or phrase in each pair that contains a shortened stop in a doubled context. Then transcribe each word.

Utterance A	Utterance B	Transcription A	Transcription B
ribbing	rib bone		
midday	middle		
lamppost	opposite		
sledding	sled down		
cottage	cattail		
subbasement	rabbit		
adopt	adduct		
crab bite	crabby		
Let Tom.	lettuce		
Stop it.	Stop Pete.		

7–18. Stops: Identifying Phrases With Glottal Stop Insertions

Circle the phrases that contain a glottal stop insertion between the vowels that end the first word and begin the second word.

roma apple	excellent ale	angry alligator
audio effect	icy icicle	her heir
busy alley	aqua sky	shy ape
edible egg	my aide	bumpy avocado
enter eagerly	azalea aroma	heavy axle

7–19. Stops: Identifying and Transcribing Words With Omission of /t/ in Word-Medial /nt/-Clusters

Circle the words for which the /t/ can be omitted in the word-medial /nt/-clusters. Then transcribe each word.

Word	Transcription
cantaloupe	_____
daughter	_____
caterpillar	_____
antibiotic	_____
interesting	_____
guitar	_____
tomato	_____
twenty	_____
beautiful	_____
plentiful	_____
computer	_____
hospital	_____
winter	_____
vegetable	_____
antonym	_____
bountiful	_____
calculator	_____
internet	_____
entrance	_____

7–20. Fricatives: Transcribing Phrases With Palatalized /s/ and /z/

Use narrow transcription to transcribe the following words, all of which can be palatalized.

Phrase	Transcription
city's youth	_____
was young	_____
plus you	_____
lose yourself	_____
girls yearn	_____
less yarn	_____
this year	_____
egg's yolk	_____
cars yield	_____
use yeast	_____
says yes	_____
his yoyo	_____
the cab's yellow	_____
Skip's yogurt	_____

7–21. Fricatives: Identifying Utterances With Devoicing of [v] in /v/ + Voiceless Consonant Contexts

Circle the phrases for which the devoicing of [v] in /v/ + voiceless consonant contexts rule can apply.

have fun	behave yourself	wave hello
arrive late	love phonetics	five trees
give thanks	move quickly	save face
dive shallow	pave streets	drive far
above board	shave carefully	believe now
remove doubt	thrive today	festive party
improve now	twelve boys	live free

7–22. Fricatives: Identifying and Transcribing Words With Voiced [s] in Voiced Consonant + /s/ Contexts

Say each word aloud, paying attention to voicing of [s] in voiced consonant + /s/ contexts. Circle the words containing voiced [s] (that is, [z]). Then transcribe each word.

Word A	Word B	Transcription A	Transcription B
pats	pans	_____	_____
dogs	dots	_____	_____
harms	hearths	_____	_____
jobs	jocks	_____	_____
wicks	whims	_____	_____
falls	faults	_____	_____
buys	bites	_____	_____
heats	heeds	_____	_____
woks	watches	_____	_____
foals	folks	_____	_____

7–23. Fricatives: Identifying and Transcribing Words With Fricative Lengthening

Say each utterance aloud, paying attention to whether both fricatives in doubled contexts are lengthened. Circle the utterances containing fricative lengthening. Then transcribe each word.

Utterance A	Utterance B	Transcription A	Transcription B
caffeine	calf feed		
his zipper	unzip		
guesser	yes sir		
buff feet	buffy		
buses	bus seat		
cat's skills	Catskills		
stuff fell	stuffing		
alphabet	half phase		
password	misspell		
graffiti	graph fuel		

7–24. Fricatives: Identifying Phrases With Omission of /h/ in Unstressed Contexts

Circle the phrases that can contain omission of /h/ in unstressed contexts.

Let's have FUN!   Look him in the EYES.

HE's a jolly good fellow.   WHICH way did he go?

PLEASE, give me her number.   Do YOU know who's going?

YOU have to HELP me.   We HAD to run fast.

I like HER attitude.   See how much it COSTS.

7–25. Affricates: Identifying and Transcribing Words With Labialized Affricates

Say each word aloud, paying attention to whether the affricate preceding the vowel is labialized rule can apply. Circle the words containing a labialized affricate. Then transcribe each word.

Word   Transcription

choke   _____

cheek   _____

chew   _____

jive   _____

juice   _____

jaw   _____

matches   _____

nachos   _____

ketchup   _____

pitcher   _____

major   _____

apologize   _____

soldier   _____

7–26. Nasals: Identifying and Transcribing Utterances With Labiodentalized /m/

1. Circle the utterances for which the labiodentalized /m/ rule can apply.

ham for dinner	some flowers	amphitheater
phone family	emphasize	swam fast
ephemeral	swim fast	palm fronds
harrumph	same friends	triumphant
film violence	from Venus	broken vase

2. All the following words can contain a labiodentalized /m/. Transcribe each word.

symphonic   _____

camphor   _____

amphibian   _____

emphatic   _____

Humvee   _____

circumvent   _____

7–27. Nasals: Identifying and Transcribing Words With Velarized /n/

Read the following sets of words aloud, paying attention to whether the *n* sounds are produced as /n/, /ŋ/, or /ŋk/. Then transcribe each word.

thin	_____	think	_____	thing	_____
sin	_____	sink	_____	sing	_____
win	_____	wink	_____	wing	_____
ran	_____	rank	_____	rang	_____
clan	_____	clank	_____	clang	_____
stun	_____	stunk	_____	stung	_____
tan	_____	tank	_____	tang	_____
angel	_____	ankle	_____	angle	_____
tongue	_____	singing	_____		
blanket	_____	thinking	_____		
trinket	_____	unkind	_____		
hanger	_____	angelic	_____		

7–28. Nasals: Identifying and Transcribing Utterances With Nasal Lengthening

Say each utterance aloud, paying attention to whether both nasals in doubled contexts are lengthened. Circle the utterances containing nasal lengthening. Then transcribe each utterance.

Utterance A	Utterance B	Transcription A	Transcription B
hammered	from Mars		
swim meet	swimmer		
running	Run now.		
unplanned	openness		
unnerve	announce		
brownnoser	annex		
summer	some money		
unnatural	penny		
tenderness	thinness		
nonnative	annihilate		

7–29. Nasals: Identifying and Transcribing Words With Syllabic Nasals

Pay attention to whether the word-final nasal is syllabic. Circle the words containing syllabic nasals. Then transcribe each word.

Word	Transcription
awaken	_____
Amazon	_____
summon	_____
magazine	_____
explain	_____
urban	_____
imprison	_____
listen	_____
ma'am	_____
burden	_____
prism	_____
column	_____

7–30. Nasals: Identifying and Transcribing Words With Nasal Lengthening and Syllabification

Say each word aloud to determine if there is evidence of nasal lengthening and/or nasal syllabification. Phonetically transcribe each word. Mark an X in the appropriate box. Then describe the reason for this type of assimilation. The first one has been done for you.

Word	Phonetic Transcription	Syllabic	Lengthened	Description
mission	ˈmɪ.ʃn̩	X		The weak vowel can be eliminated and replaced by a syllabic consonant, which acts as the nucleus of the syllable.
evenness				
rhythm				
important				
roommate				
indeed				
team mascot				

7–31. Approximants: Transcribing Words With Dark-l in Post-Vocalic Contexts

Each of the following words contains a dark-l in post-vocalic position. Transcribe each word.

<u>Word</u>   <u>Transcription</u>

fault   _____

coal   _____

film   _____

wilt   _____

mail   _____

bells   _____

guilt   _____

chalk   _____

elm   _____

soil   _____

7–32. Approximants: Identifying and Transcribing Words With Devoiced /w, j, l, ɹ/ in Voiceless Stop + Approximant Clusters

Circle the words containing a devoiced approximant as a result of the voiceless stop + approximant clusters rule. Then transcribe each word.

Word A	Word B	Transcription A	Transcription B
pew	beauty		
pajamas	pupil		
apply	apple		
plaid	bladder		
beetle	between		
dry	try		
matron	matter		
acquire	squire		
aghast	acute		
cyclops	blot		
acrid	grand		

7–33. Approximants: Identifying Phrases With Lengthened /l/

Circle the phrases that typically contain lengthening of /l/ in double /l/ contexts.

pearl locket	pal around	goal line
pencil lines	mole hill	tell her
full laundry	girl laughing	football locker
bill due	pal around	tall ladder
grill out	pole vaulter	small lock
sell land	heavy lifting	live life

7–34. Approximants: Identifying and Transcribing Words With Syllabic /l/ in Unstressed Word-Final Contexts

Circle the words for which the final /l/ can be syllabified in unstressed word-final contexts. Then transcribe each word.

Word	Transcription
final	_____
nickel	_____
bottle	_____
jackal	_____
needle	_____
hill	_____
finial	_____
peel	_____
silt	_____
saddle	_____
shelf	_____

7–35. Narrow Transcription of Sentences

Apply as many diacritics as you can to narrowly transcribe the following sentences!

Sentence   Transcription

1. The cats scattered. _____

2. Please tell the truth. _____

3. Do you want the cute puppy? _____

4. The garden died last winter. _____

5. Escape cold weather today. _____

VOWEL PHONOLOGY

8–1. Identifying and Transcribing Stressed and Unstressed Schwa and Wedge

Each of the following highlighted words has at least one vowel produced with a schwa and/or a wedge. Underline the syllable (or syllables) that contain a wedge or a schwa. Put a check in the appropriate column if the word contains a schwa, wedge, or a schwa and a wedge. Then transcribe the word, marking the stressed vowel with an apostrophe at the beginning of the syllable.

	Word	/ʌ/	/ə/	Phonetic Transcription
1.	salami			
2.	buffalo			
3.	enough			
4.	detect			
5.	between			
6.	united			
7.	televise			
8.	sunny			
9.	pumice			
10.	customary			

8–2. Identifying Schwa /ə/ and Wedge /ʌ/

For each of the following highlighted words, use the table to mark with an "X" which of the target words contains a schwa /ə/, wedge /ʌ/, both, or neither. Then transcribe the word.

Target Word	Wedge	Schwa	Both	Neither	Transcription
muffin					
can					
bucket					
malice					
luck					
unique					
above					
beauty					
forest					
stomach					
syringe					
none					
mend					
love					
summit					
cup					
data					
divide					
oven					
cut					

Target Word	Wedge	Schwa	Both	Neither	Transcription
emphasize					
puppet					
sash					
muddy					
cupboard					
sofa					
troops					
adore					

8–3. Identifying Stressed and Unstressed Vowels: /ʌ/ and /ə/

Each of the following words contain the wedge /ʌ/or the schwa /ə/. Circle the words that are most frequently produced with the unstressed schwa /ə/.

bunny	tub	jacket
bug	ocean	cut
sofa	fun	passion
dumb	shun	ability
come	about	cup
love	ago	token
silent	bus	system
plunge	reason	harmony
parrot	bottom	luck
welcome	done	rut

8–4. Transcribing Mid Central Vowel Stressed and Unstressed Allophonic Variations

Transcribe each highlighted multisyllabic word, capturing production differences of the mid central vowel with [ʌ] or [ə].

1. umbrella   _____

2. mud   _____

3. tongue   _____

4. complete   _____

5. donut   _____

6. what   _____

7. rough   _____

8. deduced   _____

9. welcome   _____

10. lunch   _____

11. rusty   _____

12. alone   _____

13. done   _____

14. provide   _____

15. plumbing   _____

16. describe   _____

8–5. Identifying and Transcribing Stressed and Unstressed Schwar

Each word has at least one vowel produced with stressed or unstressed schwar. Say the highlighted multisyllabic words aloud. Circle the syllable (or syllables) that contains a stressed or unstressed schwar. Put a check in the appropriate column if the word contains a stressed shwar, an unstressed schwar, or a stressed and an unstressed schwar. Then transcribe the word.

	Word	/ɝ/	/ɚ/	Phonetic Transcription
1.	surprise			
2.	runner			
3.	burning			
4.	stuttered			
5.	thunder			
6.	courteous			
7.	purple			
8.	furry			
9.	forgiveness			
10.	customer			

8–6. Vowel Nasalization

Circle the following words that contain a nasalized vowel.

window	thing	arithmetic
alarm	bean	hammer
potato	crown	mouth
ring	adult	pillow
tongue	nose	computer
bookcase	storm	river
drum	kidney	moon

8–7. Vowel Tenseness

Circle the words that contain a lax vowel.

cat	sit	boot
bell	hook	pond
nut	comb	tin
bet	sock	mouse
watch	sand	nail
beard	dress	push

8–8. Capturing Vowel Length

In each of the following word pairs, circle the word with the longer vowel according to rules for vowel length in English. Transcribe both words using narrow transcription and diacritics to capture the vowel length difference.

Word Pair		Narrow Transcription	
safe	save		
lock	log		
see	seating		
two	tool		
beat	bead		
set	settle		
team	tea		
cab	cap		

8–9. Vowel Length

Circle the word in each word pair that, according to typical phonological patterns of English, will contain a longer vowel.

suit	sued
play	plate
pea	peak
bit	bitter
trapper	trap
bet	bed
row	wrote
plot	dog
joy	void
shook	should

8–10. Vowel Length in Stressed Versus Unstressed Syllables

The following words are presented in pairs. Transcribe both words. A syllable in each word contains the same phonemes. Circle the word where the matching syllable would be longer. If the syllables will be the same length, circle both words. Remember that for /ʌ/ and /ɝ/, stress distinctions can be captured with allophonic symbols [ə] and [ɚ].

1. fasten   sunny   _____   _____

2. into   intact   _____   _____

3. catsup   bobcat   _____   _____

4. current   recur   _____   _____

5. delete   athlete   _____   _____

6. coughing   finger   _____   _____

7. urbane   purring   _____   _____

8. admit   summit   _____   _____

9. gulping   beagle   _____   _____

10. support   portly   _____   _____

8–11. Vowel Length

Put the following words in order based on length of vowel production in each of them (longest to shortest). Assume the only difference in vowel length is based on English phonological patterns.

/i/	knead	sheet	bee	mosquito

/ɪ/	ability	bigger	kiss	dig

/ʊ/	neighborhood	put	should	rookie

/aɪ/	type	excite	bye	excitement

/u/	January	computer	views	compute

/e/	state	bathe	locate	location

/ɛ/	net	education	red	better

/aʊ/	cloud	cow	flower	shout

/oʊ/	roam	show	devote	soap

/ʌ/	independence	alert	tub	summer

8–12. Coarticulation

For each word in the following chart, describe in detail the type of anticipatory and/or carryover coarticulation that will likely occur on the vowel. Then transcribe the word, using narrow transcription to capture the coarticulation.

Word	Description	Narrow Transcription
1. spoon		
2. basketball		
3. install		
4. architect		
5. tropical		
6. rebel		
7. sprain		
8. wrong		
9. win		
10. still		

8–13. Transcription Errors

Which of the following transcriptions contain an error? Mark C for correct and I for incorrect. If incorrect, transcribe the word correctly.

chapter	t͡ʃæpdɚ	_____	_____
grain	ɡɹe͡ɪn	_____	_____
push	pʊʃ	_____	_____
plate	ple͡ɪt	_____	_____
desk	dɛsk	_____	_____
boat	bo͡ʊt	_____	_____
phone	fɔn	_____	_____
dot	dat	_____	_____
rain	ɹæn	_____	_____
pie	pi	_____	_____
boy	bɔ͡ɪ	_____	_____
cloud	klo͡ʊd	_____	_____
bird	bɝd	_____	_____
leaf	lɛf	_____	_____
mop	mɑp	_____	_____
feel	fil	_____	_____
sun	sən	_____	_____
kit	kɪt	_____	_____
bus	bʌs	_____	_____
rat	ɹɑt	_____	_____

8–14. Diacritic Use

Each of the following words contain a diacritic providing additional information about the vowel. Circle "correct" if the diacritic correctly describes General American English vowel phonological patterns. Circle "incorrect" if the diacritic is not used correctly.

stɹi̩t	Correct	Incorrect
dɹĩŋk	Correct	Incorrect
tɹiː	Correct	Incorrect
ˈbɑ̩.ɹəl	Correct	Incorrect
ˈwʊ.mẽn	Correct	Incorrect
ˈpɛn.sə̥ɫ	Correct	Incorrect
hɪ̩ɫ	Correct	Incorrect
ˈpæ.kə̃t	Correct	Incorrect
bɹɪ̩k	Correct	Incorrect

8–15. Identifying Accurate Narrow Transcription

Circle the best narrow transcription of the following words.

1.	topography	tʰə.ˈpʰɑ̩.gɹə.fi	tʰə̩.ˈpʰɑ.gɹə.fi	tʰə.ˈpʰɑ.gɹə.fi̥
2.	sheet	ʃi̩tˈ	ʃi̩tˈ	ʃi̩tˈ
3.	name	nei̩m	nei̩m	nẽɪm
4.	telephone	ˈtʰɛ.lə.foõn	ˈtʰɛ.lə.foõn	ˈtɛ.lə̩.foŏn
5.	feel	fi̩ɫ	fĩl	fĩl
6.	potato	pʰə.ˈtʰeɪ.ɾoʊ	pʰə.ˈtʰeɪ.ɾo̥ʊ	pʰə̩.ˈtʰeɪ.ɾoʊ
7.	monkey	ˈmɑ̃ŋ.kʰi	ˈmʌ̩ŋ.kʰĩ	ˈmʌ̩ŋ.kʰi
8.	shadow	ˈʃæʰ.ɾoʊ	ˈʃæ.ɾoʊ	ˈʃæ.ɾoʊ
9.	catastrophe	kʰə.ˈtʰæ.stɹə.fi	kʰə̩.ˈtʰæ.stɹə.fi̥	kʰə̩.ˈtʰæ.stɹə.fi
10.	ring	ɹĩŋ	ɹi̩ŋ	ɹi̩ŋ
11.	track	tɹ̥æk	tɹ̥æk	tɹæk
12.	drip	dɹɪʷp	dɹɪ̈p	dɹɪ̩p

8–16. Narrow Transcription

Say aloud. Transcribe the highlighted words, using diacritics to differentiate vowel length and vowel stress patterns.

listen _____

currently _____

attitude _____

council _____

obvious _____

union _____

again _____

impossible _____

downhill _____

musical _____

persuasive _____

another _____

education _____

destroying _____

mathematics _____

communication _____

9

BEYOND GENERAL AMERICAN ENGLISH
Speech Possibilities Within and Across Languages

9–1. Language Terms

Complete the following definitions with the correct term.

1. A person who uses more than two languages is called a _____

2. Mutually intelligible variants of a language are called _____

3. The predecessor of all languages in a language family is a _____

4. Related languages that share linguistic properties belong to a(n) _____

5. A person who uses two languages is called a(n) _____

6. A language used by people to communicate when they do not share the same first language is called a(n) _____.

7. A community's shared communication of words and rules for combining and producing words is called a(n) _____.

8. Dialects that trace back to a geographic region are called _____.

9. Dialects that are shared by individuals identifying as a subgroup of a community are called _____.

9–2. Identifying Active and Passive Articulators

Determine if the following places of articulation are active or passive and upper or lower surface.

1. Tongue front   _____

2. Hard palate   _____

3. Alveolar ridge   _____

4. Tongue root   _____

5. Lower lip   _____

6. Pharyngeal wall   _____

7. Post-alveolar region   _____

8. Soft palate   _____

9. Tongue back   _____

10. Tongue blade   _____

11. Underside of the tongue   _____

12. Upper lip   _____

13. Uvula   _____

14. Tongue tip   _____

9–3. Identifying Pulmonic Consonants

Circle yes or no to indicate whether the place, manner, and voicing combinations are phonemic in English. Transcribe the phoneme.

		Phonemic in English?	Phonetic Transcription
1.	voiced uvular stop	Yes / No	_____
2.	voiced labiodental nasal	Yes / No	_____
3.	voiced dental fricative	Yes / No	_____
4.	voiceless glottal stop	Yes / No	_____
5.	voiced bilabial trill	Yes / No	_____
6.	voiced retroflex flap	Yes / No	_____
7.	voiceless palatal stop	Yes / No	_____
8.	voiced lateral palatal liquid	Yes / No	_____
9.	voiceless velar fricative	Yes / No	_____
10.	voiced palatal fricative	Yes / No	_____
11.	voiced palatal approximant glide	Yes / No	_____
12.	voiced uvular nasal	Yes / No	_____

9–4. Airstream Terminology

Complete the following definitions with the correct term.

1. If a speech sound is produced when air is leaving the vocal tract, it is produced on an
   _____ airstream.

2. If a speech sound is produced when air is rushing into the vocal tract, it is produced on
   an _____ airstream.

3. The airstream source for a click is _____

4. The airstream source for an ejective is _____

5. The airstream source for a plosive is _____

6. A speech sound made on a velaric ingressive airstream is called a(n) _____

7. A speech sound made on a glottalic egressive airstream is called a(n) _____

8. A speech sound made on a pulmonic egressive airstream is called a(n) _____

9. A speech sound made on a glottalic ingressive airstream is called a(n) _____

9–5. Airstreams Used in Speech Production

Which airstream source and direction is used to make each of the following sounds?

1. Click   _____

2. Ejective   _____

3. Nasal   _____

4. Plosive   _____

5. Fricative   _____

6. Implosive   _____

7. Vowel   _____

8. Liquid   _____

9–6. Non-Pulmonic Sounds

Write the articulatory characterizations for the following non-pulmonic IPA symbols (voicing, place, and manner). An example has been done for you.

1. /ǃk/   <u>voiceless postalveolar click</u>

2. /ǂŋ/   _____

3. /p'/   _____

4. /ǀk/   _____

5. /ʘg/   _____

6. /ʙ/   _____

7. /ʜ/   _____

8. /ɗ/   _____

9. /t'/   _____

10. /β/   _____

11. /ʄ/   _____

12. /ʐ/   _____

13. /ɬ/   _____

14. /ǁg/   _____

9–7. Airflow

Identify whether each phoneme has an egressive or ingressive airflow. Circle the correct answer.

1. /k'/   a) ingressive   b) egressive

2. /ɓ/   a) ingressive   b) egressive

3. /m/   a) ingressive   b) egressive

4. /ʘg/   a) ingressive   b) egressive

5. /ɢ/   a) ingressive   b) egressive

6. /s'/   a) ingressive   b) egressive

7. /w/   a) ingressive   b) egressive

8. /ǂŋ/   a) ingressive   b) egressive

9. /ɗ/   a) ingressive   b) egressive

10. /ǃk/   a) ingressive   b) egressive

9–8. Describing and Contrasting Sounds Across Languages

The following times indicate different voice onset time (VOT) delays. Match these possible VOT delays with the type of plosive consonant.

                    –20 ms   0 ms   40 ms   80 ms

Strongly aspirated stop   _____

Voiceless unaspirated stop   _____

Fully voiced stop   _____

Slightly aspirated stop   _____

9–9. Describing Consonants

You were introduced to nine ways that consonants can differ. These are (1) airstream source, (2) airstream direction, (3) state of glottis, (4) part of tongue (can be NA), (5) place, (6) centrality, (7) nasality, (8) manner, and (9) length. Define the nine categories for each of the following sounds.

1. /p'/
1) _____ 2) _____ 3) _____
4) _____ 5) _____ 6) _____
7) _____ 8) _____ 9) _____

2. /‖ŋ/
1) _____ 2) _____ 3) _____
4) _____ 5) _____ 6) _____
7) _____ 8) _____ 9) _____

3. /ʄː/
1) _____ 2) _____ 3) _____
4) _____ 5) _____ 6) _____
7) _____ 8) _____ 9) _____

4. /ɢ/
1) _____ 2) _____ 3) _____
4) _____ 5) _____ 6) _____
7) _____ 8) _____ 9) _____

5. /ḏ/
1) _____ 2) _____ 3) _____
4) _____ 5) _____ 6) _____
7) _____ 8) _____ 9) _____

6. /ʙː/
1) _____ 2) _____ 3) _____
4) _____ 5) _____ 6) _____
7) _____ 8) _____ 9) _____

7. / l̪ /
1) _____ 2) _____ 3) _____
4) _____ 5) _____ 6) _____
7) _____ 8) _____ 9) _____

8. /t͡s'/   1) _____   2) _____   3) _____

4) _____   5) _____   6) _____

7) _____   8) _____   9) _____

9–10. Speech Sound Inventories

The following are contrived vowel and consonant inventories for different languages. Note whether these inventories are likely or unlikely and why.

1. Language A Vowels: /i, ɪ, y, ʏ, ɛ, e, æ/

_____

_____

_____

2. Language B Vowels: /i, e, ɑ, o, u/

_____

_____

_____

3. Language C Vowels: /i, ẹ, a͡ɪ, õ, uː/

_____

_____

_____

4. Language D Vowels: /i, e, ɛ/

_____

_____

_____

5. Language A Consonants: /N, ʕ, ʀ, ʐ, ʟ/

_____

_____

_____

6. Language B Consonants: /d, g, b, m, n, s, f, j/

_____

_____

_____

TRANSCRIPTION PRACTICE

10–1. Single-Syllable Words: 1

1. *back* _____

2. *time* _____

3. *jump* _____

4. *rogue* _____

5. *shield* _____

6. *tone* _____

7. *breathe* _____

8. *church* _____

9. *guest* _____

10. *bathe* _____

11. *hook* _____

12. *globe* _____

10–2. Single-Syllable Words: 2

1. *think*   _____

2. *scream*   _____

3. *down*   _____

4. *oak*   _____

5. *beef*   _____

6. *shake*   _____

7. *missed*   _____

8. *beige*   _____

9. *sheep*   _____

10. *lunch*   _____

11. *smooth*   _____

12. *count*   _____

10–3. Single-Syllable Words: 3

1. *date*   _____

2. *curb*   _____

3. *eat*   _____

4. *cheese*   _____

5. *few*   _____

6. *this*   _____

7. *was*   _____

8. *yolk*   _____

9. *vowel*   _____

10. *zest*   _____

11. *blaze*   _____

12. *shine*   _____

10–4. Single-Syllable Words: 4

1. *thank*   _____

2. *dwell*   _____

3. *reach*   _____

4. *yard*   _____

5. *trust*   _____

6. *mesh*   _____

7. *dish*   _____

8. *fly*   _____

9. *shut*   _____

10. *boot*   _____

11. *moon*   _____

12. *theft*   _____

10–5. Single-Syllable Words: 5

1. *month* _____

2. *sign* _____

3. *latch* _____

4. *shrink* _____

5. *zoo* _____

6. *booth* _____

7. *those* _____

8. *theft* _____

9. *shrimp* _____

10. *ledge* _____

11. *stretch* _____

12. *wait* _____

10–6. Single-Syllable Words: 6

1. *boss*   _____

2. *spring*   _____

3. *vague*   _____

4. *they*   _____

5. *soft*   _____

6. *tongue*   _____

7. *splash*   _____

8. *squirrel*   _____

9. *buzz*   _____

10. *caught*   _____

11. *sign*   _____

12. *who*   _____

10–7. Single-Syllable Words: 7

1. *use*   _____

2. *vine*   _____

3. *sixths*   _____

4. *treat*   _____

5. *cloth*   _____

6. *fair*   _____

7. *cut*   _____

8. *day*   _____

9. *chin*   _____

10. *egg*   _____

11. *the*   _____

12. *five*   _____

10–8. Single-Syllable Words: 8

1. *age*   _____

2. *camp*   _____

3. *good*   _____

4. *bill*   _____

5. *not*   _____

6. *razed*   _____

7. *fun*   _____

8. *breath*   _____

9. *seen*   _____

10. *tough*   _____

11. *threw*   _____

12. *key*   _____

10–9. Single-Syllable Words: 9

1. *sick*   _____

2. *glass*   _____

3. *shop*   _____

4. *groove*   _____

5. *hat*   _____

6. *he*   _____

7. *in*   _____

8. *jazz*   _____

9. *kite*   _____

10. *straw*   _____

11. *wake*   _____

12. *tie*   _____

10–10. Single-Syllable Words: 10

1. *lose*   _____

2. *miss*   _____

3. *name*   _____

4. *bait*   _____

5. *cat*   _____

6. *pill*   _____

7. *nice*   _____

8. *crush*   _____

9. *each*   _____

10. *this*   _____

11. *staff*   _____

12. *yes*   _____

10–11. Single-Syllable Words: 11

1. *hopped* _____

2. *oath* _____

3. *pack* _____

4. *gifts* _____

5. *robe* _____

6. *pry* _____

7. *push* _____

8. *bath* _____

9. *geese* _____

10. *read* _____

11. *time* _____

12. *rock* _____

10–12. Single-Syllable Words: 12

1. *dwarf*   _____

2. *see*   _____

3. *ghost*   _____

4. *leaf*   _____

5. *chain*   _____

6. *lift*   _____

7. *rope*   _____

8. *which*   _____

9. *vine*   _____

10. *date*   _____

11. *sun*   _____

12. *team*   _____

10–13. Single-Syllable Words: 13

1. *strength* _____

2. *that* _____

3. *might* _____

4. *wish* _____

5. *cough* _____

6. *maps* _____

7. *cute* _____

8. *did* _____

9. *nest* _____

10. *this* _____

11. *knee* _____

12. *threat* _____

10–14. Multisyllabic Words: 1

1. *giant* _____

2. *nephew* _____

3. *rather* _____

4. *fishing* _____

5. *backache* _____

6. *about* _____

7. *giggling* _____

8. *jacket* _____

9. *kangaroo* _____

10. *recent* _____

11. *adore* _____

12. *singer* _____

10–15. Multisyllabic Words: 2

1. *bacon* _____

2. *hammer* _____

3. *summer* _____

4. *royal* _____

5. *behold* _____

6. *advantage* _____

7. *hanger* _____

8. *bachelor* _____

9. *kitchen* _____

10. *calming* _____

11. *lodges* _____

12. *again* _____

10–16. Multisyllabic Words: 3

1. *higher*   _____

2. *bother*   _____

3. *mahogany*   _____

4. *unit*   _____

5. *ginger*   _____

6. *collage*   _____

7. *terrible*   _____

8. *agitate*   _____

9. *story*   _____

10. *casual*   _____

11. *otter*   _____

12. *number*   _____

10–17. Multisyllabic Words: 4

1. *along* _____

2. *music* _____

3. *vision* _____

4. *city* _____

5. *beacon* _____

6. *office* _____

7. *anger* _____

8. *dizzy* _____

9. *blanket* _____

10. *October* _____

11. *anyhow* _____

12. *coughing* _____

10–18. Multisyllabic Words: 5

1. *banana* _____

2. *occasion* _____

3. *peaches* _____

4. *carrot* _____

5. *before* _____

6. *eerie* _____

7. *anything* _____

8. *easy* _____

9. *somebody* _____

10. *either* _____

11. *ribbon* _____

12. *pretty* _____

10–19. Multisyllabic Words: 6

1. *aphasia* _____

2. *zodiac* _____

3. *profit* _____

4. *usual* _____

5. *ripen* _____

6. *family* _____

7. *stopping* _____

8. *toothbrush* _____

9. *coffee* _____

10. *single* _____

11. *weather* _____

12. *potato* _____

10–20. Multisyllabic Words: 7

1. *envious*   _____

2. *bucket*   _____

3. *stocking*   _____

4. *burrito*   _____

5. *fasten*   _____

6. *prestige*   _____

7. *visit*   _____

8. *feather*   _____

9. *ashamed*   _____

10. *lesson*   _____

11. *fashion*   _____

12. *gentle*   _____

10–21. Multisyllabic Words: 8

1. *value* _____

2. *begin* _____

3. *peanut* _____

4. *Athens* _____

5. *magic* _____

6. *orange* _____

7. *possible* _____

8. *servant* _____

9. *widen* _____

10. *ego* _____

11. *wealthy* _____

12. *treasure* _____

10–22. Multisyllabic Words: 9

1. *virtue* _____

2. *basin* _____

3. *voyage* _____

4. *breathy* _____

5. *cathedral* _____

6. *yellow* _____

7. *believe* _____

8. *wishes* _____

9. *rehearse* _____

10. *dollar* _____

11. *earthquake* _____

12. *father* _____

10–23. Multisyllabic Words: 10

1. *happy*   _____

2. *jelly*   _____

3. *kitten*   _____

4. *loyal*   _____

5. *mother*   _____

6. *nation*   _____

7. *obvious*   _____

8. *bigger*   _____

9. *oppose*   _____

10. *pebble*   _____

11. *dozen*   _____

12. *camouflage*   _____

10–24. Short Phrases: 1

1. *black cat*

2. *hot water*

3. *poster board*

4. *yellow ladder*

5. *purple paint*

6. *icy pavement*

7. *galloping horse*

8. *take care*

9. *early riser*

10. *crowded buses*

11. *phonetic transcription*

12. *communication disorder*

10–25. Short Phrases: 2

1. *rotating disks* _____

2. *devoted students* _____

3. *eager beaver* _____

4. *auditory processing* _____

5. *migraine headache* _____

6. *bouncing baby* _____

7. *chocolate cheesecake* _____

8. *Caribbean cruise* _____

9. *destroyed building* _____

10. *one toothbrush* _____

11. *measuring cups* _____

12. *happy birthday* _____

10–26. Longer Phrases: 1

1. *fabulous mosaic*   _____

2. *talking chatterbox*   _____

3. *playing the harp*   _____

4. *elephants in pajamas*   _____

5. *fudge mint Oreos*   _____

6. *azure ocean blue*   _____

7. *ladies and gentlemen*   _____

8. *bagels or strudel*   _____

9. *going skiing*   _____

10. *ticket's booked*   _____

11. *person of wealth*   _____

12. *cheddar cheese quesadillas* _____

10–27. Longer Phrases: 2

1. *brown paper packages* _____

2. *gigantic eighteen wheeler* _____

3. *Californian abstract artist* _____

4. *professor of audiology* _____

5. *sprint up the hill* _____

6. *colorful impressionist painting* _____

7. *flexible Olympic gymnast* _____

8. *bright blossoming sunflower* _____

9. *triangles, squares, rectangles* _____

10. *remembering childhood daydreams* _____

11. *rambunctious kindergarteners* _____

12. *delicious huckleberry pie* _____

10–28. Sentences: 1

1. *Please fasten your seatbelts.*

   _____

2. *I'd like to order the vegetable souffle.*

   _____

3. *Five o'clock is rush hour.*

   _____

4. *She is certain it's not pouring.*

   _____

5. *My favorite movie is Jurassic Park.*

   _____

6. *She went to her high school reunion.*

   _____

7. *He wore a tuxedo with shiny black shoes.*

   _____

8. *The garden is overflowing with shrubs and bushes.*

   _____

9. *Spaghetti is a delicious meal.*

   _____

10. *Don't be noisy or you'll get in trouble.*

    _____

11. *Leopard print is back in fashion.*

    _____

12. *Turn up the stereo, so I can hear the music.*

    _____

10–29. Sentences: 2

1. *Report the theft to the state police.*

_____

2. *Study hard and you will succeed.*

_____

3. *He plays the electric guitar.*

_____

4. *My friend sews floral pillowcases.*

_____

5. *The record player has broken again.*

_____

6. *Store leftovers in plastic containers.*

_____

7. *Stop talking while I'm watching the television.*

_____

8. *Consonants are either voiced or voiceless.*

_____

9. *Chocolate brownies with marshmallow sauce taste good.*

_____

10. *Be nice to all the teacher's assistants.*

_____

11. *Can I borrow a pencil?*

_____

12. *My chores take hours to finish.*

_____

10–30. Sentences: 3

1. *The flowers are pretty.*

_____

2. *There is a bird in that tree.*

_____

3. *The child's singing is lovely.*

_____

4. *Raindrops are falling from the sky.*

_____

5. *My sister is a judge on the Supreme Court.*

_____

6. *Did you study for the test?*

_____

7. *In the winter, I like to ski with my friends and family.*

_____

8. *Will you come to my birthday party on Friday?*

_____

9. *He is the fastest racer.*

_____

10. *I will meet you there in one hour to work on the group project.*

_____

11. *She sells seashells by the seashore.*

_____

12. *I scream, you scream, we all scream for ice cream.*

_____

10–31. Sentences: 4

1. *Put the books away.*

_____

2. *Two young boys are looking for their toys.*

_____

3. *I love the music on this tour.*

_____

4. *Wish upon a star.*

_____

5. *Let's go see a movie.*

_____

6. *Where are you from?*

_____

7. *I've heard so much about you.*

_____

8. *The rabbit got out of his cage and now he is missing.*

_____

9. *It's so good to see you again.*

_____

10. *Tourists like to go whale watching when they visit the coast.*

_____

11. *What time does the bus arrive?*

_____

12. *Thank you for giving me a ride to the airport in the middle of the night.*

_____

10–32. Sentences: 5

1. *It is important to measure ingredients when baking.*

_____

2. *There are a lot of fish swimming upstream this time of year.*

_____

3. *Where is the nearest hospital?*

_____

4. *Do not touch service dogs when they are working.*

_____

5. *She can read and write very well for her age.*

_____

6. *Kids often forget their jackets at school.*

_____

7. *The rose garden is growing nicely this year.*

_____

8. *His dream is to be a homeowner.*

_____

9. *You will need a bow and arrows for your first archery lesson.*

_____

10. *Jack loves to go camping during spring break.*

_____

11. *She is graduating from high school in June.*

_____

12. *My cousin will be visiting us in the summer.*

_____

ANSWER KEY

INTRODUCTION TO PHONETIC SCIENCE

1–1. Branches of Phonetics

Indicate which branch of phonetics is being practiced in each scenario: articulatory, acoustic, auditory, or linguistic.

1. Determining if a *z* sound changes in spectral frequency over time by examining a speech spectrogram (a spectrogram is a visible representation of speech).
    acoustic

2. Determining if a child's tongue tip is raised or lowered when they produce an *s* sound by watching the child's mouth during speech production.
    articulatory

3. Determining if a child is transferring a sound pattern from their native language to words in their second language by examining a written transcript of the words they said.
    linguistic

4. Determining if a bilingual adult can differentiate between two sounds—one sound in their native language and one sound in a language they do not speak.
    auditory

5. Determining if the vocal folds vibrate during production of the *v* sound by feeling the laryngeal area during production.
    articulatory

6. Determining lip movement during production of *b* in word-final position.
    articulatory

7. Determining that *t* and *g* encode meaning in English because the words *"dot"* and *"dog"* are different words.
    linguistic

8. Determining the average vocal pitch of French-speaking children.
   acoustic

9. Determining if a grade-school child can tell the difference between sounds produced using the tip of the tongue.
   auditory

10. Determining that the *th* sound is meaningful in English but not in German.
    linguistic

1–2. Phonemes and Phones

Read each pair of phrases. Place each phrase that denotes the concept of phonemes between virgules, and place the phrases that denote the concept of phones between brackets. The first pair has been done for you.

phonemes   /phonemes/

phones   [phones]

planning or production of speech sounds   **[planning or production of speech sounds]**
mental representations of speech sounds   **/mental representations of speech sounds/**

the word   /**the word**/
the word spoken   [**the word spoken**]

the thought of producing a word   [**thinking of how a word is produced**]
the thought of a word   /**the thought of a word**/

language   /**language**/
speech   [**speech**]

out of the mouth   [**out of the mouth**]
in the head   /**in the head**/

1–3. The Continuum of Archaic to Intimate Speech Registers

A. Write the following sentences to represent **citation-form** speech.

1. Why ain'tcha goin'?
   Why aren't you going?

2. Where ya been?
   Where have you been?

3. I gotta git movin'.
   I have to get moving.

4. She sumpm else!
   She is something else!

5. Howdja do on the test?
   How did you do on the test?

B. Write the following sentences to represent **casual** speech.

1. Can you believe it?
   Can ya b'lieve it?

2. I really want a day off.
   I really wanna day off.

3. What did you buy?
   Whatcha buy?

4. I would love to see you again!
   I'd love ta see ya 'gain!

5. Let me help you with that.
   Lemme help ya widat.

C. Fill in the following blanks. Then practice reading the paragraph aloud to someone using citation-form speech. Be clear and precise in your articulation, but avoid extreme overexaggeration. Ask your listener for feedback on your articulation. Then, think about how it felt to produce citation-form speech and to whom and in what situations would you speak using a formal or consultative register.

Answers will vary.

Hello! My name is _____ and I am very happy to meet you. I am originally from _____, and I have been living in _____ for the past _____. I am studying phonetics because _____ _____. One thing I already have learned in phonetics that I find interesting is _____.

1. Describe the feedback you received from your listener.

_____

_____

_____

_____

_____

2. Note how it felt producing formal speech.

_____

_____

_____

_____

_____

3. To whom and in what situations would you speak using a formal register?

_____

_____

_____

_____

_____

1–4. Analyzing Spoken Words: Number of Sounds and Syllables

Low Level of Difficulty

Complete the chart for the words listed.

Word	# of Sounds	# of Syllables
bat	3	1
hip-hop	6	2
is	2	1
swim	4	1
hand	4	1
sank	4	1
grand	5	1
dental	6	2
second	6	2
analysis	8	4
electron	8	3
kayak	5	2
static	6	2
pencil	6	2

Moderate Level of Difficulty

Complete the chart for the words listed.

Word	# of Sounds	# of Syllables
why	2	1
gnat	3	1
they	2	1
six	4	1
couch	3	1
thumb	3	1
known	3	1
balloon	5	2
ship	3	1
amount	5	2
right	3	1
famous	5	2
jumped	5	1
knife	3	1
success	6	2

High Level of Difficulty

Complete the chart for the words listed.

Word	# of Sounds	# of Syllables
beauty	5	2
extension	9	3
refuse	6	2
language	7	2
spatula	7	3
exhaust	6	2
suggestion	9	3
rhythm	5	2
castle	5	2
reputation	10	4
studying	8	3
vicarious	8	4
earthquake	6	2
ambitious	7	3
ubiquitous	10	4

1–5. Analyzing Spoken Words: Phonotactic Structure and Syllabicity

Low Level of Difficulty

Complete the chart for the words listed.

Word	Phonotactic Structure	Syllabicity
bat	CVC	CVC
hip-hop	CVCCVC	CVC.CVC
is	VC	VC
swim	CCVC	CCVC
hand	CVCC	CVCC
sank	CVCC	CVCC
grand	CCVCC	CCVCC
dental	CVCCVC	CVC.CVC
second	CVCVCC	CV.CVCC
analysis	VCVCVCVC	V.CV.CV.CVC
electron	VCVCCCVC	V.CVC.CCVC
kayak	CVCVC	CV.CVC
static	CCVCVC	CCV.CVC
pencil	CVCCVC	CVC.CVC

Moderate Level of Difficulty

Complete the chart for the words listed.

Word	Phonotactic Structure	Syllabicity
why	CV	CV
gnat	CVC	CVC
they	CV	CV
six	CVCC	CVCC
couch	CVC	CVC
thumb	CVC	CVC
known	CVC	CVC
balloon	CVCVC	CV.CVC
ship	CVC	CVC
amount	VCVCC	V.CVCC
right	CVC	CVC
famous	CVCVC	CV.CVC
jumped	CVCCC	CVCCC
knife	CVC	CVC
success	CVCCVC	CVC.CVC

High Level of Difficulty

Complete the chart for the words listed.

Word	Phonotactic Structure	Syllabicity
beauty	CCVCV	CCV.CV
extension	VCCCVCCVC	VC.CCVC.CVC
refuse	CVCCVC	CV.CCVC
language	CVCCCVC	CVC.CCVC
spatula	CCVCVCV	CCV.CV.CV
exhaust	VCCVCC	VC.CVCC
suggestion	CVCCVCCVC	CVC.CVC.CVC
rhythm	CVCVC	CV.CVC
castle	CVCVC	CV.CVC
reputation	CVCCVCVCVC	CVC.CV.CV.CVC
studying	CCVCVCVC	CCV.CV.CVC
vicarious	CVCVCVCVC	CV.CV.CV.VC
earthquake	VCCCVC	VC.CCVC
ambitious	VCCVCVC	VC.CV.CVC
ubiquitous	CVCVCCVCVC	CV.CV.CCV.CVC

1–6. Analyzing Spoken Words: Position of Consonants in Words

Complete the chart for the words listed. Leave blank any cells without data.

Word	Word-Initial Position	Word-Medial Position	Word-Final Position
bat	b		t
is			z
swim	sw		m
hand	h		nd
second	s	c	nd
avoid		v	d
static	st	t	c
pencil	p	nc	l
thumb	th		m
balloon	b	l	n
knife	n		f
beauty	bj	t	
exhaust		gz	st
suggest	s	gj	st
rhythm	r	th	m
castle	c	s	l
stringy	str	ng	

1–7. Analyzing Spoken Words: Position of Consonants in Syllables

Complete the chart for the words listed. Leave blank any cells without data.

Word	Syllable-1 Initial Position	Syllable-1 Final Position	Syllable-2 Initial Position	Syllable-2 Final Position
bat	b	t		
is		z		
swim	sw	m		
hand	h	nd		
second	s		c	nd
avoid			v	d
static	st		t	c
pencil	p	n	c	l
thumb	th	m		
balloon	b		l	n
knife	n	f		
beauty	bj		t	
exhaust		g	z	st
suggest	s	g	j	st
rhythm	r		th	m
castle	c		s	l
stringy	str	ng		

1–8. Analyzing Spoken Words: Identifying the Stressed Syllable

For each word, indicate the syllable that is stressed. The first word has been done as an example.

Word	Stressed Syllable
dental	syllable 1
second	syllable 1
analysis	syllable 2
electron	syllable 2
kayak	syllable 1
static	syllable 1
pencil	syllable 1
balloon	syllable 2
amount	syllable 2
famous	syllable 1
jumped	syllable 1
success	syllable 2
beauty	syllable 1
extension	syllable 2
language	syllable 1
spatula	syllable 1
exhaust	syllable 2
suggestion	syllable 2
rhythm	syllable 1
castle	syllable 1
reputation	syllable 3
studying	syllable 1
vicarious	syllable 2
earthquake	syllable 1
ambitious	syllable 2
ubiquitous	syllable 2

ARTICULATORY PHONETICS: CONSONANTS

2–1. Writing Phonetic Consonant Symbols

Practice drawing each phonetic symbol several times on the line.

Name	Phonetic Symbol	Practice
eng	ŋ	
theta	θ	
ethe	ð	
esh	ʃ	
ezh	ʒ	
tesh digraph	t͡ʃ	
dezh digraph	d͡ʒ	
turned R	ɹ	

2–2. Matching Phonetic Symbols to Alphabet Letters

Match each phonetic symbol in the left-hand column with its corresponding alphabet letter(s) in the right-hand column.

1. k   (j)   a.   th (as in *thigh*)
2. ŋ   (e)   b.   sh
3. j   (g)   c.   soft "c"
4. θ   (a)   d.   ch
5. ð   (i)   e.   ng (as in *sing*)
6. s   (c)   f.   j (as in *jay*)
7. ʃ   (b)   g.   y
8. t͡ʃ   (d)   h.   r
9. d͡ʒ   (f)   i.   th (as in *thy*)
10. ɹ   (h)   j.   hard "c" (as in *candy*)

2–3. Identifying Voiced and Voiceless Consonant Phonemes in Isolation

Indicate if each consonant represents a sound that is voiced or voiceless.

1. p   voiced – **voiceless**
2. d   **voiced** – voiceless
3. k   voiced – **voiceless**
4. ɹ   **voiced** – voiceless
5. ʒ   **voiced** – voiceless
6. w   **voiced** – voiceless
7. f   voiced – **voiceless**
8. ð   **voiced** – voiceless
9. z   **voiced** – voiceless

10. h   voiced – **voiceless**

11. d͡ʒ   **voiced** – voiceless

12. l   **voiced** – voiceless

2–4. Identifying Voiced and Voiceless Consonant Phonemes in Words

Indicate whether each bolded consonant (or consonants) represents a phoneme that is voiced or voiceless.

1. b as in *boo*   **voiced** – voiceless

2. t as in *too*   voiced – **voiceless**

3. g as in *goo*   **voiced** – voiceless

4. m as in *moo*   **voiced** – voiceless

5. j as in *you*   **voiced** – voiceless

6. v as in *voodoo*   **voiced** – voiceless

7. θ as in *through*   voiced – **voiceless**

8. s as in *sue*   voiced – **voiceless**

9. ʃ as in *shoe*   voiced – **voiceless**

10. t͡ʃ as in *chew*   voiced – **voiceless**

11. ɹ as in *rue*   **voiced** – voiceless

12. f as in *flew*   voiced – **voiceless**

2–5. Matching Phonetic Consonant Symbols to Articulatory Place

Match each phonetic symbol with its place of articulation.

1. z   (d)   a. bilabial

2. j   (g)   b. labiodental

3. h   (i)   c. interdental

4. f   (b)   d. alveolar

5. ð   (c)   e. post-alveolar

6. w   (a)   f. alveopalatal

7. d͡ʒ   (f)   g. palatal

8. ŋ   (h)   h. velar

9. ʃ   (e)   i. glottal

2–6. Matching Phonetic Consonant Symbols to Articulatory Place

Match each phonetic symbol with the appropriate place of articulation.

1. ʒ   (d)   a. labiodental

2. h   (h)   b. interdental

3. t͡ʃ   (e)   c. alveolar

4. ɹ   (f)   d. post-alveolar

5. m   (i)   e. alveopalatal

6. k   (g)   f. palatal

7. θ   (b)   g. velar

8. v   (a)   h. glottal

9. t   (c)   i. bilabial

2–7. Matching Phonetic Consonant Symbols to Manner Class

Match each individual or pair of phonetic symbols with the appropriate manner of articulation.

1. ʃ **(d)**	a.	stop
2. d͡ʒ **(e)**	b.	nasal
3. l **(f)**	c.	glide
4. d **(a)**	d.	fricative
5. w, ɹ **(g)**	e.	affricate
6. n **(b)**	f.	liquid
7. w **(c)**	g.	approximant

2–8. Matching Phonetic Consonant Symbols to Manner Class

Match each individual or pair of phonetic symbols to the appropriate manner of articulation.

1. j **(c)**	a.	stop
2. h **(d)**	b.	nasal
3. t͡ʃ **(e)**	c.	glide
4. k **(a)**	d.	fricative
5. ɹ **(f)**	e.	affricate
6. m **(b)**	f.	liquid

2–9. Describing Consonantal Articulation

Fill in the missing information.

Alphabetic Letter(s)	Phonetic Symbol	Voiced (+) or Voiceless (–)	Place of Articulation	Manner of Articulation
p	p	–	bilabial	stop
d	d	+	alveolar	stop
g	g	+	velar	stop
n	n	+	alveolar	nasal
ng	ŋ	+	velar	nasal
y	j	+	palatal	glide
v	v	+	labiodental	fricative
s	s	–	alveolar	fricative
sh	ʃ	–	post-alveolar	fricative
h	h	–	glottal	fricative
j	d͡ʒ	+	alveopalatal	affricate
r	ɹ	+	palatal	liquid

2–10. Describing Consonant Sounds in Words

Fill in the missing information for the bolded sound in each word.

Sound in Word	Phonetic Symbol	Word-Initial, Word-Medial, or Word-Final Position	Voiced (+) or Voiceless (–)	Place of Articulation	Manner of Articulation
bet	b	initial	+	bilabial	stop
be**t**	t	final	–	alveolar	stop
catch	k	initial	–	velar	stop
cat**ch**	t͡ʃ	final	–	alveopalatal	affricate
woman	w	initial	+	bilabial	glide
wo**m**an	m	medial	+	bilabial	nasal
ba**th**	θ	final	–	interdental	fricative
ba**th**e	ð	final	+	interdental	fricative
e**ss**ay	s	medial	–	alveolar	fricative
ea**s**y	z	medial	+	alveolar	fricative
fa**ll**ing	l	medial	+	alveolar	liquid
falli**ng**	ŋ	final	+	velar	nasal

2–11. What Consonant Am I?

Determine the consonant phoneme(s) described by each clue.

1. I am a voiced bilabial glide.   /w/

2. I am a voiceless alveolar stop.   /t/

3. I am a voiceless post-alveolar fricative.   /ʃ/

4. I am a voiced velar stop.   /g/

5. I am a voiceless glottal fricative.   /h/

6. I am a voiced interdental fricative.   /ð/

7. I am a voiced retroflex liquid.   /ɹ/

8. I am a pair of alveolar fricatives.   /s, z/

9. I am a voiced alveopalatal affricate.   /d͡ʒ/

10. I am a voiced velar nasal.   /ŋ/

11. I am a voiced palatal glide.   /j/

12. I am a voiceless bilabial stop.   /p/

13. I am a voiceless alveolar fricative.   /s/

14. I am a pair of labiodental fricatives.   /f, v/

15. I am the cognate of /ð/.   /θ/

2–12. What Am I?

Read the clues to guess the word described.

1. I have a voiced alveolar stop in word-initial position.

    I turn into the crust of a pizza when baked.

    I am made of flour and tossed into the air.

    What am I?   _____ **dough** _____

2. I have a voiced bilabial stop in word-medial position.

    I am a piece of furniture.

    I am surrounded by chairs.

    What am I?   _____ **table** _____

3. I have a voiceless velar stop in word-final position.

    I have words written inside of me.

    I can make you laugh or cry or even become smarter.

    What am I?   _____ **book** _____

4. I have a voiced bilabial nasal in word-initial position.

I am used to purchase things.

I am currency.

What am I?   _____*money*_____

5. I have a voiced velar nasal in word-medial position.

I am used to keep clothes off the floor.

I am made of wood, plastic, or metal.

What am I?   _____*hanger*_____

6. I have a voiced alveolar nasal in word-final position.

I am used to write on paper.

I have ink.

What am I?   _____*pen*_____

7. I have a voiced bilabial glide in word-medial position.

I look and smell nice.

I can be bought in a bouquet.

What am I?   _____*flower*_____

8. I have a voiced palatal glide in word-initial and word-medial positions.

I am a round toy you hold in your hand, and I have a long string to move me up and down.

Rock the baby, anyone?

What am I?   _____*yo-yo*_____

9. I have a voiced labiodental fricative in word-initial position.

I am a decorative container.

I am made of glass, wood, or plastic.

What am I?   _____*vase*_____

10. I have a voiceless interdental fricative in word-initial position.

I am found on an extremity.

I am the opposable digit.

What am I?   _____**thumb**_____

11. I have a voiceless alveolar fricative in word-medial position.

I am a toddler eating spaghetti and meatballs with my fingers.

I am a child eating an ice cream cone on a hot summer day.

What am I?   _____**messy**_____

12. I have a voiceless glottal fricative in word-medial position.

I am a popular internet search engine.

I also am an expression that usually is said with enthusiasm!

What am I?   _____**yahoo**_____

13. I have a voiced alveopalatal affricate in word-initial position.

I am the place you go to work every day.

I am where you earn a living.

What am I?   _____**job**_____

14. I have a voiceless alveopalatal affricate in word-final position.

I am what you strike to make fire.

I come in a pack.

What am I?   _____**match**_____

15. I have a voiced palatal liquid in word-initial position.

I am the color of a Valentine's heart.

I am the color of blood.

What am I?   _____**red**_____

16. I have a voiced alveolar liquid in word-medial position.

I am a depth of water.

I am not deep.

What am I?   _____**shallow**_____

2–13. Building Words

Build words of the following phonotactic shapes using the designated consonants.

> First, let's do one for practice: CVbV. Remember to focus on the sounds in words, not the orthographic letters.
>
> What words might work for this pattern? Would *ruby, maybe, tube,* and *knobby* work?
>
> The word *ruby* would work. It has four sounds: consonant sound [ɹ], long vowel sound "u," target consonant [b], and long vowel sound "e."
>
> The word *maybe* would work too. It also has four sounds: consonant sound [m], long vowel sound "a," target sound [b], and long vowel sound "e."
>
> The word *tube* would not work, even though it's spelled with four consonant-vowel-consonant-vowel letters, because the word *tube* has only three sounds: consonant sound [t], long vowel sound "u," and target sound [b]. The final letter "e" is silent.
>
> Last, the word *knobby* would work. There are four sounds in *knobby*: consonant sound [n], vowel sound "ah," target consonant [b], and long vowel sound "e."

1. CVpV   *happy, mopey, sippy,* and so forth

2. bVbV   *baby, Bobby, Bobo,* and so forth

3. CVt   *cat, dot, sheet,* and so forth

4. dVd   *dad, dude, died,* and so forth

5. kCVC   *crag, clock, quack,* etc.

6. CVg   *bag, hog, thug,* and so forth

7. CVmVC   *demon, roaming, hammock,* and so forth

8. CVCVn   *taken, button, tighten,* and so forth

9. CVŋVŋ   *singing, banging, wronging,* and so forth

10. wVC   *wit, watch, wait,* and so forth

11. jVjV   *yoyo*

12. VfCVC   *often, offset, Aflac,* and so forth

13. VvVC   *oven, evil, oval,* and so forth

14. CVθ   *bath, mouth, myth,* and so forth

15. CVð   *bathe, soothe, teethe,* and so forth

16. sCCVC   *strap, stripe, straight,* and so forth

17. CVz   *buzz, has, Ms.,* and so forth

18. CVʃVC   *washing, lotion, dishes,* and so forth

19. ʒVC   none in English!

20. VhV   *ahoy, aha, oho,* and so forth

21. CVt͡ʃ   *much, beach, patch,* and so forth

22. d͡ʒVd͡ʒ   *judge*

23. CVlV   *lily, jolly, valley,* and so forth

24. ɹVCVC   *running, writing, raucous,* and so forth

ARTICULATORY PHONETICS: VOWELS

3–1. Hearing Vowel Phonemes

Read the words for each question aloud. Listen carefully to the vowels. One word in each question has a different vowel phoneme. Circle the word with the differing vowel.

1.	book	should	**hide**	pull
2.	bead	sneak	**said**	cheese
3.	rid	fish	hitch	**raw**
4.	say	pail	trace	**top**
5.	**aunt**	kept	chest	bread
6.	cad	**code**	badge	bath
7.	**couch**	heart	marked	barn
8.	hood	cook	**caught**	push
9.	toe	snow	**hot**	ghost
10.	who	**here**	cruise	flew
11.	sir	**snarl**	search	curve
12.	**man**	tide	hive	sign
13.	how	loud	**book**	bough
14.	toy	boy	**lone**	coil
15.	sneer	**tend**	pier	beard
16.	**dear**	hair	chaired	prayer
17.	squire	**tip**	tires	higher
18.	cower	**choir**	sours	floured

3–2. Identifying Monophthong Vowel Phonemes in Orthographic Transcription

/i/

/i/ is the vowel in *bee, keen,* and *sea.* Circle which of the following words contain /i/.

soul	**tree**	pen	**seize**
heal	try	play	quit
dine	focus	**queen**	sigh
case	fly	cat	wash

/ɪ/

/ɪ/ is the vowel in *bit, kick,* and *chin.* Circle which of the following words contain /ɪ/.

speech	quite	mop	**mint**
heal	**hymn**	play	**slit**
dine	bear	loud	sigh
last	eel	**squid**	**kit**

/e/ - [eɪ]

[eɪ] is the frequent production of /e/ in *say, case,* and *late.* Circle which of the following words contain [eɪ].

feel	tree	**vain**	**makes**
heal	try	**play**	lamp
dine	**bane**	**quail**	**chase**
quake	**phase**	crab	blessed

/ɛ/

/ɛ/ is the vowel in *let, well,* and *gem.* Circle which of the following words contain /ɛ/.

case	tree	**stench**	choice
shell	mount	play	quit
knot	**head**	**felt**	traipse
now	goat	cat	beat

/æ/

/æ/ is the vowel in *bat, fast,* and *sack.* Circle which of the following words contain /æ/.

dough	baste	vain	**trap**
mop	spout	**plaque**	strength
ban	mouse	**last**	dozen
tree	case	**thatch**	say

/ʌ/

/ʌ/ is the vowel in *sun, just,* and *tuck.* Circle which of the following words contain /ʌ/.

bath	**dug**	end	**fudge**
goat	try	hurt	**none**
cut	**bug**	last	sigh
love	case	cough	**strut**

/ɝ/

/ɝ/ is the vowel in *shirt, burn,* and *her.* Circle which of the following words contain /ɝ/.

duck	**fern**	core	best
man	fire	**church**	swear
squirrel	twin	roar	**surge**
lark	fun	**work**	tired

/u/

/u/ is the vowel in *new, shoe,* and *pool.* Circle which of the following words contain /u/.

punt	**blue**	**booth**	mean
moon	brand	play	hall
strut	burn	**choose**	**suit**
who	fly	**drew**	book

/ʊ/

/ʊ/ is the vowel in *cook, would,* and *hood.* Circle which of the following words contain /ʊ/.

brood	budge	food	**puts**
rush	case	**foot**	squashed
dine	**book**	trend	**pushed**
could	try	first	last

/o/ - [o͡ʊ]

[o͡ʊ] is the typical production of /o/ in *low, go,* and *soak.* Circle which of the following words contain [o͡ʊ].

show	bond	**goat**	**bone**
hand	**toast**	spout	quit
broke	doubt	leaf	thought
mean	crowd	**dough**	posh

/ɔ/

/ɔ/ is the vowel in *log, saw,* and *thought.* Circle which of the following words contain /ɔ/. If you don't have /ɔ/ in your lexicon, circle the words that have /a/.

pool	put	dug	**bought**
whole	try	dough	**hall**
thaw	doze	trap	sigh
spout	case	envy	last

/a/

/a/ is the vowel in *hot, sock,* and *fall.* Circle which of the following words contain /a/.

dine	enemy	**watt**	mean
cot	bad	play	quit
fly	**mop**	eel	case
knot	**shot**	trash	**mom**

3–3. Identifying Diphthong Vowel Phonemes in Orthographic Transcription

/aɪ/

/aɪ/ is the vowel in *fly, dime,* and *tie.* Circle which of the following words contain /aɪ/.

cried	**vine**	mean	psalm
heal	**try**	play	soup
dine	more	**find**	**sigh**
screech	case	skate	beat

/aʊ/

/aʊ/ is the vowel in *cow, shout,* and *ounce.* Circle which of the following words contain /aʊ/.

louse	**now**	friend	maze
feed	try	**spout**	**mound**
dine	books	splay	flipped
chair	**crowd**	glass	**slouch**

/ɔɪ/

/ɔɪ/ is the vowel in *boy, soil,* and *joy.* Circle which of the following words contain /ɔɪ/.

point	now	chips	mar
loud	**choice**	try	quit
dine	wolf	**oil**	**toy**
moist	shirt	cat	though

3–4. Identifying Rhotic Diphthongs and Triphthongs in Orthographic Transcription

/ɪɚ/

/ɪɚ/ is the vowel in *fear, cheered,* and *steers.* Circle which of the following words contain /ɪɚ/.

flirt	point	nor	**fierce**
clear	**spheres**	trees	quit
dine	bear	coin	**year**
wire	shirt	**beard**	cares

/ɛ͡ɚ/

/ɛ͡ɚ/ is the vowel in *bear, shared,* and *hair.* Circle which of the following words contain /ɛ͡ɚ/.

brash	cars	door	**bared**
tires	**dare**	**rare**	score
fair	brown	pliers	twist
moored	brawn	sure	**blare**

/ʊ͡ɚ/

/ʊ͡ɚ/ is the vowel in *cured* and *manure.* Circle which of the following words can contain /ʊ͡ɚ/. If this vowel phoneme is not in your lexicon, circle the words where you could produce [ʊ͡ɚ]

chord	**tour**	vent	bite
lure	bathe	**cure**	shard
toil	fjord	rear	chew

/ɔ͡ɚ/

/ɔ͡ɚ/ is the vowel in *boar, corn,* and *fort.* Circle which of the following words contain /ɔ͡ɚ/.

post	**born**	kale	pushed
glove	choice	worked	**scorn**
course	drive	look	plot
soar	worse	cat	**quart**

/ɑ͡ɚ/

/ɑ͡ɚ/ is the vowel in *barn, charge,* and *art.* Circle which of the following words contain /ɑ͡ɚ/.

swatch	spot	chai	**farm**
loud	**chard**	stork	**spark**
learn	boor	**snarl**	turn
coil	shirt	bush	bare

/aɪɚ/

/aɪɚ/ is the vowel in *ire, dryer,* and *briar.* Circle which of the following words contain /aɪɚ/.

cried	slow	board	parse
laud	thrice	**dire**	poor
dive	bear	oil	**tire**
hoist	**higher**	**spire**	roar

/aʊɚ/

/aʊɚ/ is the vowel in *our, showers,* and *powered.* Circle which of the following words contain /aʊɚ/.

cower	now	dirge	**dour**
loud	plaque	**flour**	lock
dine	bear	oil	tour
fire	shirt	**tower**	joke

3–5. Shared Vowel Phoneme

For each of the following questions, read the list of words aloud to yourself. You'll notice that one of the words in the list has a different vowel phoneme than the other words. Cross out the word that contains a different vowel. Add a word that shares the vowel phoneme of the remaining words.

1.	eight	~~that~~	shade	change	answers will differ
2.	coat	~~down~~	hope	post	answers will differ
3.	time	right	bite	~~make~~	answers will differ
4.	lap	tap	~~neck~~	wag	answers will differ
5.	cook	~~shoot~~	foot	hook	answers will differ
6.	steep	~~check~~	neat	sheep	answers will differ
7.	luck	hut	bug	~~chute~~	answers will differ
8.	pig	~~bike~~	hip	trim	answers will differ
9.	~~row~~	mouth	foul	vow	answers will differ
10.	botch	~~joy~~	rot	shop	answers will differ

3–6. Determining Type of Vowel

Tongue Advancement

Indicate whether each vowel is front, central, or back.

1. ʌ   front   **central**   back

2. e͡ɪ   **front**   central   back

3. ɪ   **front**   central   back

4. æ   **front**   central   back

5. ɛ   **front**   central   back

6. ɔ   front   central   **back**

7. ɝ   front   **central**   back

8. u   front   central   **back**

9. ʊ   front   central   **back**

10. i   **front**   central   back

Tongue Height

Indicate whether each vowel is high, mid, or low.

1. ɑ   high   mid   **low**

2. ʊ   **high**   mid   low

3. ʌ   high   **mid**   low

4. ɝ   high   **mid**   low

5. i   **high**   mid   low

6. ɛ   high   **mid**   low

7. æ   high   mid   **low**

8. u   **high**   mid   low

9. ɪ   **high**   mid   low

10. ɔ   high   **mid**   low

Lip Rounding

Indicate whether each vowel is rounded or unrounded.

1. ɑ   rounded   **unrounded**

2. ʊ   **rounded**   unrounded

3. ʌ   rounded   **unrounded**

4. ɝ   **rounded**   unrounded

5. i   rounded   **unrounded**

6. ɛ   rounded   **unrounded**

7. æ   rounded   **unrounded**

8. u   **rounded**   unrounded

9. ɪ   rounded   **unrounded**

10. ɔ   **rounded**   unrounded

3–7. Phonetic Transcription to English Orthographic Spelling

Read the following words. Write the English word that represents the phonemic transcription. There are three examples of each English vowel, including rhotic vowels.

1. a. /it/   **eat**
   b. /bif/   **beef**
   c. /wik/   **week / weak**

2. a. /kɑp/   **cop**
   b. /ʃɑk/   **shock**
   c. /sɑb/   **sob**

3. a. /fɪʃ/   **fish**
   b. /wɪt͡ʃ/   **which / witch**
   c. /θɪŋk/   **think**

4. a. /d͡ʒɛt/   **jet**
   b. /ʃɛd/   **shed**
   c. /tɛst/   **test**

5.   a.   /gæs/   **gas**

    b.   /bæθ/   **bath**

    c.   /ðæt/   **that**

6.   a.   /stʌk/   **stuck**

    b.   /bʌnt͡ʃ/   **bunch**

    c.   /d͡ʒʌŋk/   **junk**

7.   a.   /d͡ʒɝm/   **germ**

    b.   /ʃɝt/   **shirt**

    c.   /pɝt͡ʃ/   **perch**

8.   a.   /tuθ/   **tooth**

    b.   /t͡ʃuz/   **choose**

    c.   /gus/   **goose**

9.   a.   /gʊd/   **good**

    b.   /kʊk/   **cook**

    c.   /hʊd/   **hood**

10.   a.   /kɔt/   **caught**

    b.   /ɹɔt/   **wrought**

    c.   /bɔt/   **bought**

11.   a.   /sket/   **skate**

    b.   /wed͡ʒ/   **wage**

    c.   /beʒ/   **beige**

12.   a.   /ɹot/   **wrote / rote**

    b.   /ston/   **stone**

    c.   /ðoz/   **those**

13.   a.   /ka͡ɪt/   **kite**

    b.   /ta͡ɪp/   **type**

    c.   /sa͡ɪn/   **sign / sine**

14. a. /vɔɪd/   **void**

   b. /plɔɪ/   **ploy**

   c. /d͡ʒɔɪ/   **joy**

15. a. /sau̯θ/   **south**

   b. /dɹau̯t/   **drought**

   c. /kau̯t͡ʃ/   **couch**

16. a. /jɪɚz/   **years**

   b. /klɪɚ/   **clear**

   c. /bɪɚd/   **beard**

17. a. /ʃɛɚ/   **share**

   b. /skwɛɚ/   **square**

   c. /t͡ʃɛɚz/   **chairs**

18. a. /kjʊɚ/   **cure**

   b. /pjʊɚ/   **pure**

   c. /tʊɚd/   **toured**

19. a. /bɔɚd/   **bored**

   b. /flɔɚ/   **floor**

   c. /hɔɚs/   **horse**

20. a. /ʃɑɚp/   **sharp**

   b. /dɑɚk/   **dark**

   c. /d͡ʒɑɚ/   **jar**

21. a. /taɪɚd/   **tired**

   b. /waɪɚ/   **wire**

   c. /plaɪɚz/   **pliers**

22. a. /au̯ɚ/   **hour / our**

   b. /sau̯ɚ/   **sour**

   c. /skau̯ɚd/   **scoured**

3–8. Phonetic Transcription of Vowels

Practice writing the symbols for the vowels in the following words.

Sound	IPA Symbol	Transcription Practice
f<u>ee</u>t	i	
k<u>i</u>t	ɪ	
c<u>a</u>se	e͡ɪ	
br<u>ea</u>d	ɛ	
c<u>a</u>t	æ	
b<u>u</u>g	ʌ	
b<u>ir</u>d	ɝ	
f<u>oo</u>d	u	
t<u>oo</u>k	ʊ	
b<u>oa</u>t	o͡ʊ	
c<u>augh</u>t	ɔ	
h<u>o</u>t	ɑ	
s<u>igh</u>	a͡ɪ	
t<u>oy</u>	ɔ͡ɪ	
<u>ou</u>t	a͡ʊ	
f<u>ear</u>	i͡ɚ	
c<u>are</u>	ɛ͡ɚ	
t<u>our</u>	ʊ͡ɚ	
ch<u>ore</u>	ɔ͡ɚ	
t<u>ar</u>	ɑ͡ɚ	
h<u>ire</u>	a͡ɪɚ	
<u>our</u>	a͡ʊɚ	

3–9. Learning Vowel Descriptive Categories

Transcribe the following words using the International Phonetic Alphabet (IPA). You'll need to use the vowel symbols you have learned in Chapter 3 as well as the English consonant symbols you learned in Chapter 2.

Once you have transcribed the word, describe the vowel by each characteristic that applies. The first one has been done for you.

		Transcription	High, Mid, or Low?	Front, Central, or Back?	Lax or Tense?	Rounded or Unrounded?
1.	ask	æsk	low	front	lax	unrounded
2.	end	ɛnd	mid	front	lax	unrounded
3.	ill	ɪl	high	front	lax	unrounded
4.	geese	gis	high	front	tense	unrounded
5.	stew	stu	high	back	tense	rounded
6.	shook	ʃʊk	high	back	lax	rounded
7.	hug	hʌg	mid	central	lax	unrounded
8.	soap	so͡up - sop	mid	back	tense	rounded
9.	dock	dɑk	low	back	tense	unrounded
10.	bit	bɪt	high	front	lax	unrounded
11.	read	ɹid	high	front	tense	unrounded
12.	melt	mɛlt	mid	front	lax	unrounded
13.	pass	pæs	low	front	lax	unrounded
14.	cruise	kɹuz	high	back	tense	rounded
15.	bush	bʊʃ	high	back	lax	rounded
16.	bus	bʌs	mid	central	lax	unrounded
17.	fox	fɑks	low	back	tense	unrounded
18.	deep	dip	high	front	tense	unrounded
19.	kick	kɪk	high	front	lax	unrounded

		Transcription	High, Mid, or Low?	Front, Central, or Back?	Lax or Tense?	Rounded or Unrounded?
20.	deck	dɛk	mid	front	lax	unrounded
21.	perk	pɝk	mid	central	tense	rounded
22.	gum	gʌm	mid	central	lax	unrounded
23.	face	feɪs - fes	mid	front	tense	unrounded
24.	book	bʊk	high	back	lax	rounded
25.	knock	nɑk	low	back	tense	unrounded
26.	brook	bɹʊk	high	back	lax	rounded
27.	run	ɹʌn	mid	central	lax	unrounded
28.	lewd	lud	high	back	tense	rounded
29.	elk	ɛlk	mid	front	lax	unrounded
30.	peel	pil	high	front	tense	unrounded

3–10. Shared Categories

Each of the following questions has three vowel phonemes listed. These three vowel phonemes share a common property. Please explain how the three vowels are alike.

1. /i/   /u/   /ʊ/   **high vowels**

2. /ɑ/   /u/   /i/   **tense vowels**

3. /æ/   /ɪ/   /ɑ/   **unrounded vowels**

4. /aɪ/   /ɪɚ/   /ɔɪ/   **(phonemic) diphthongs**

5. /ʊ/   /ɝ/   /ɔ/   **rounded vowels**

6. /i/   /ɛ/   /e/   **front vowels**

7. /ɛ/   /ɔ/   /ʌ/   **mid vowels**

8. /ɛ/   /ʊ/   /ɪ/   **lax vowels**

9. /o/   /ʊ/   /ɑ/   **back vowels**

10. /aɪɚ/   /ɝ/   /ɪɚ/   **rhotic vowels**

3–11. Discover the Vowel

Determine the vowel and the referenced word with the following information.

1. /b/ + high back vowel + /t/   Vowel: /u/   Word: **boot**

2. /ɪ/ + mid central vowel + /f/   Vowel: /ʌ/   Word: **rough**

3. /p/ + low central diphthong +/t͡ʃ/   Vowel: /a͡ʊ/   Word: **pouch**

4. /b/ + low front vowel + /θ/   Vowel: /æ/   Word: **bath**

5. /ʃ/ + mid front vowel + /v/   Vowel: /e/   Word: **shave**

6. /d͡ʒ/ + mid back vowel + /k/   Vowel: /o/   Word: **joke**

7. /f/ + low back vowel + /l/   Vowel: /ɑ/   Word: **fall**

8. /t͡ʃ/ + mid front vowel + /k/   Vowel: /ɛ/   Word: **check**

9. /d͡ʒ/ + mid back diphthong + /n/   Vowel: /ɔ͡ɪ/   Word: **join**

10. /t/ + high front vowel + /p/   Vowel: /ɪ/   Word: **tip**

3–12. How Many Phonemes?

Count the phonemes in each of the following words. Hint: It will be easier to count phonemes if you transcribe each word before you get started.

1. frown   4   /fɹa͡ʊn/

2. brake   4   /bɹe͡ɪk/ - /bɹek/

3. jail   3   /d͡ʒe͡ɪl/ - /d͡ʒel/

4. scrunched   7   /skɹʌnt͡ʃt/

5. wrath   3   /ɹæθ/

6. friend   5   /fɹɛnd/

7. muse   4   /mjuz/

8. changed   5   /t͡ʃe͡ɪnd͡ʒd/

9. hope   3   /ho͡ʊp/

10. comb   3   /ko͡ʊm/

11. things   4   /θɪŋz/

12. brook   4   /bɹʊk/

13. feet   3   /fit/

14. shorts   4   /ʃɔɚts/

3–13. English Orthographic Spelling to Phonetic Transcription

Phonetically transcribe the following English words. The words are organized by vowel phoneme.

1. Words containing the high front tense unrounded vowel /i/.

   east **ist**   tree **tɹi**   neat **nit**   sheep **ʃip**   cheek **t͡ʃik**

2. Words containing the high front lax unrounded vowel /ɪ/.

   tip **tɪp**   thick **θɪk**   lit **lɪt**   mist **mɪst**   fridge **fɹɪd͡ʒ**

3. Words containing the mid front to high front tense unrounded nonphonemic diphthong [eɪ].

   snake **sneɪk**   they **ðeɪ**   cape **keɪp**   glaze **gleɪz**   cage **keɪd͡ʒ**

4. Words containing the mid front lax unrounded vowel /ɛ/.

   stem **stɛm**   shed **ʃɛd**   jet **d͡ʒɛt**   them **ðɛm**   best **bɛst**

5. Words containing the low front lax unrounded vowel /æ/.

   batch **bæt͡ʃ**   flap **flæp**   track **tɹæk**   badge **bæd͡ʒ**   yak **jæk**

6. Words containing the mid central lax unrounded vowel /ʌ/.

   truck **tɹʌk**   dutch **dʌt͡ʃ**   sunk **sʌŋk**   fudge **fʌd͡ʒ**   young **jʌŋ**

7. Words containing the mid central tense rounded vowel /ɝ/.

   perch **pɝt͡ʃ**   surge **sɝd͡ʒ**   first **fɝst**   third **θɝd**   yearn **jɝn**

8. Words containing the high back tense rounded vowel /u/.

   cute **kjut**   boost **bust**   choose **t͡ʃuz**   fruit **fɹut**   coop **kup**

9. Words containing the high back lax rounded vowel /ʊ/.

   brook **bɹʊk**   could **kʊd**   crook **kɹʊk**   hook **hʊk**   stood **stʊd**

10. Words containing the mid back to high back rounded nonphonemic diphthong [o͡ʊ].

joke d͡ʒo͡ʊk   throat θɹo͡ʊt   ghost go͡ʊst   show ʃo͡ʊ   vote vo͡ʊt

11. Words containing the mid back to high back rounded diphthong /ɔ/.

caught kɔt   dog dɔg   flawed flɔd   taught tɔt   bought bɔt

12. Words containing the low back tense unrounded vowel /ɑ/.

yacht jɑt   shock ʃɑk   botch bɑt͡ʃ   lox lɑks   squat skwɑt

13. Words containing the low central to high front unrounded diphthong /a͡ɪ/.

bite ba͡ɪt   slide sla͡ɪd   guy ga͡ɪ   white wa͡ɪt   type ta͡ɪp

14. Words containing the mid back rounded to high front unrounded diphthong /ɔ͡ɪ/.

soil sɔ͡ɪl   joy d͡ʒɔ͡ɪ   voice vɔ͡ɪs   coin kɔ͡ɪn   choice t͡ʃɔ͡ɪs

15. Words containing the low central unrounded to high back rounded diphthong /a͡ʊ/.

doubt da͡ʊt   brown bɹa͡ʊn   cloud kla͡ʊd   shout ʃa͡ʊt   pouch pa͡ʊt͡ʃ

16. Words containing the rhotic diphthong /ɪ͡ɚ/.

jeer d͡ʒɪ͡ɚ   dear dɪ͡ɚ   beers bɪ͡ɚz   smeared smɪ͡ɚd   cheer t͡ʃɪ͡ɚ

17. Words containing the rhotic diphthong /ɛ͡ɚ/.

blare blɛ͡ɚ   airs ɛ͡ɚz   chair t͡ʃɛ͡ɚ   paired pɛ͡ɚd   square skwɛ͡ɚ

18. Words containing the rhotic diphthong /ʊ͡ɚ/.

lure lʊ͡ɚ   tour tʊ͡ɚ   pure pjʊ͡ɚ   you're jʊ͡ɚ

19. Words containing the rhotic diphthong /ɔ͡ɚ/.

quart kwɔ͡ɚt   swarm swɔ͡ɚm   thwart θwɔ͡ɚt   horse hɔ͡ɚs   court kɔ͡ɚt

20. Words containing the rhotic diphthong /ɑ͡ɚ/.

farm fɑ͡ɚm   jarred d͡ʒɑ͡ɚd   hearth hɑ͡ɚθ   charge t͡ʃɑ͡ɚd͡ʒ   start stɑ͡ɚt

21. Words containing the rhotic triphthong /a͡ɪɚ/.

pliers pla͡ɪɚz   mired ma͡ɪɚd   fire fa͡ɪɚ   friar fɹa͡ɪɚ   squire skwa͡ɪɚ

22. Words containing the rhotic diphthong /a͡ʊɚ/.

towers ta͡ʊɚz   showered ʃa͡ʊɚd   sour sa͡ʊɚ   power pa͡ʊɚ   our a͡ʊɚ

3–14. Decipher the Vowel Phoneme

Fill in the blank with the appropriate vowel symbols from the description given. Then write the word in English orthography.

1.	b___d	low, front	æ	**bad**
2.	k___t	high, front	ɪ	**kit**
3.	ʃ___t	high, back	u	**shoot**
4.	k___p	mid, central	ʌ	**cup**
5.	st___p	low, back	ɑ	**stop**
6.	k___lt	mid, back	o͡ʊ	**colt**
7.	f___t	low, central	a͡ɪ	**fight**
8.	g___n	low, central	a͡ʊ	**gown**
9.	b___g	mid, front	ɛ	**beg**
10.	t͡ʃ___f	high, front	i	**chief**

3–15. Monophthong Versus Diphthong Versus Rhotic

For each of the following words, determine if the vowel <u>phoneme</u> is a monophthong, diphthong, or rhotic. After you have circled the correct choice, phonetically transcribe the word.

1.	pit	**monophthong**	diphthong	rhotic	/pɪt/
2.	bore	monophthong	**diphthong**	**rhotic**	/bɔ͡ɚ/
3.	chat	**monophthong**	diphthong	rhotic	/t͡ʃæt/
4.	shoot	**monophthong**	diphthong	rhotic	/ʃut/
5.	owl	monophthong	**diphthong**	rhotic	/a͡ʊl/
6.	great	**monophthong**	diphthong	rhotic	/gɹet/ - [gɹe͡ɪt]
7.	down	monophthong	**diphthong**	rhotic	/da͡ʊn/
8.	peer	monophthong	**diphthong**	**rhotic**	/pɪ͡ɚ/
9.	shown	**monophthong**	diphthong	rhotic	/ʃon/ - [ʃo͡ʊn]

10.	caught	**monophthong**	diphthong	rhotic	/kɔt/ - /kɑt/
11.	teach	**monophthong**	diphthong	rhotic	/tit͡ʃ/
12.	blurt	**monophthong**	diphthong	**rhotic**	/blɝt/

3–16. What Am I?

Read the clues and guess each word described. Write the word orthographically and phonetically.

1. My vowel is a monophthong or a nonphonemic diphthong.

I am used to go from place to place quickly.

I have pilots and flight attendants on my crew.

What am I? **plane** /plen/ - [plẽɪn]

2. My vowel is a low, front monophthong.

I am used in the game of baseball.

I can be made from aluminum or wood.

What am I? **bat** /bæt/

3. My vowel is a phonemic diphthong.

I will be an adult in my future.

I like to play outside.

What am I? **child** /t͡ʃaɪld/

4. My vowel is a back diphthong.

I have a painted face and a big red nose.

I work in a circus.

What am I? **clown** /klaʊn/

5. My vowel is low and back.

I am used to keep your feet warm.

I only come in pairs.

What am I? **socks** /sɑks/

6. My vowel is a phonemic diphthong.

   I have a tail and fly in the sky.

   I am traditionally the shape of a diamond.

   What am I?   **kite**   /ka͡ɪt/

7. My vowel is a high, back monophthong.

   I am used to hold your jackets or keys.

   I am the villain from Peter Pan.

   What am I?   **hook**   /hʊk/

8. My vowel is a rhotic monophthong.

   I begin and end with bilabial stops.

   I am a rude sound made while eating.

   What am I?   **burp**   /bɝp/

BROAD AND NARROW PHONETIC TRANSCRIPTION

4–1. Accurate or Inaccurate?

Determine whether each word that follows is transcribed accurately. Circle "yes "if accurate and "no" if the transcription is inaccurate. If the transcription is incorrect, transcribe the word correctly on the line provided. Note that errors can be consonant or vowel phonemes.

1. knit   /nɪt/   Accurate: **Yes** / No

2. tough   /tɑf/   Accurate: Yes / **No**   /tʌf/

3. quest   /qwɛst/   Accurate: Yes / **No**   /kwɛst/

4. bush   /bʊʃ/   Accurate: **Yes** / No

5. sung   /sɑŋ/   Accurate: Yes / **No**   /sʌŋ/

6. bath   /bæθ/   Accurate: **Yes** / No

7. switch   /swit͡ʃ/   Accurate: Yes / **No**   /swɪt͡ʃ/

8. worm   /wɔ͡ɚm/   Accurate: Yes / **No**   /wɝm/

9. guard   /gɑ͡ɚd/   Accurate: **Yes** / No

10. wrote   /wɹo͡ʊt/   Accurate: Yes / **No**   /ɹo͡ʊt/

4–2. Phonetic Transcription: Stops, Nasals, and Glides With Front Vowels

Phonetically transcribe each word after identifying the number of phonemes in each word.

Word	# of Phonemes	Phonetic Transcription
win	3	[wɪn]
bean	3	[bin]
man	3	[mæn]
at	2	[æt]
pant	4	[pænt]
dig	3	[dɪg]
kin	3	[kɪn]
bend	4	[bɛnd]
yam	3	[jæm]
meat	3	[mit]
beat	3	[bit]
beg	3	[bɛg]
bent	4	[bɛnt]
king	3	[kɪŋ]
mend	4	[mɛnd]

4–3. Phonetic Transcription: Stops, Nasals, and Glides With Front Vowels

Phonetically transcribe each word after identifying the number of phonemes in each word.

Word	# of Phonemes	Phonetic Transcription
pat	3	[pæt]
bed	3	[bɛd]
pet	3	[pɛt]
knee	2	[ni]
bin	3	[bɪn]
mint	4	[mɪnt]
quit	4	[kwɪt]
nag	3	[næg]
bet	3	[bɛt]
be	2	[bi]
key	2	[ki]
camp	4	[kæmp]
mat	3	[mæt]
yet	3	[jɛt]
bang	3	[bæŋ]

4–4. Phonetic Transcription: Stops, Nasals, and Glides With Central and Back Vowels

Phonetically transcribe each word after identifying the number of phonemes in each word.

Word	# of Phonemes	Phonetic Transcription
nut	3	[nʌt]
boot	3	[but]
dog	3	[dɑg] - [dɔg]
book	3	[bʊk]
wand	4	[wɑnd]
took	3	[tʊk]
cough	3	[kɑf] - [kɔf]
suit	3	[sut]
not	3	[nɑt]
want	4	[wɑnt]
tug	3	[tʌg]
dot	3	[dɑt]
tong	3	[tɑŋ] - [tɔŋ]
cut	3	[kʌt]
you	2	[ju]

4–5. Phonetic Transcription: Stops, Nasals, and Glides With Central and Back Vowels

Phonetically transcribe each word after identifying the number of phonemes in each word.

Word	# of Phonemes	Phonetic Transcription
yawn	3	[jɑn] - [jɔn]
taught	3	[tɑt] - [tɔt]
what	3	[wʌt]
pun	3	[pʌn]
bump	4	[bʌmp]
gone	3	[gɑn] - [gɔn]
nook	3	[nʊk]
mood	3	[mud]
daunt	4	[dɑnt] - [dɔnt]
boo	2	[bu]
young	3	[jʌŋ]
lot	3	[lɑt]
wood	3	[wʊd]
on	2	[ɑn] - [ɔn]
doom	3	[dum]

4–6. Phonetic Transcription: Stops, Nasals, and Glides With Diphthong Vowels

Phonetically transcribe each word after identifying the number of phonemes in each word.

Word	# of Phonemes	Phonetic Transcription
mine	3	[maɪn]
wait	3	[weɪt]
boy	2	[bɔɪ]
cow	2	[kaʊ]
boat	3	[boʊt]
toe	2	[toʊ]
pain	3	[peɪn]
buy	2	[baɪ]
gaze	3	[geɪz]
time	3	[taɪm]
mount	4	[maʊnt]
coin	3	[kɔɪn]
goat	3	[goʊt]
point	4	[pɔɪnt]
town	3	[taʊn]

4–7. Phonetic Transcription: Stops, Nasals, and Glides With Diphthong Vowels

Phonetically transcribe each word after identifying the number of phonemes in each word.

Word	# of Phonemes	Phonetic Transcription
toy	2	[tɔɪ]
now	2	[naʊ]
toad	3	[toʊd]
cake	3	[keɪk]
white	3	[waɪt]
might	3	[maɪt]
dime	3	[daɪm]
out	2	[aʊt]
oink	3	[ɔɪŋk]
dome	3	[doʊm]
comb	3	[koʊm]
boink	4	[bɔɪŋk]
bang	3	[bæŋ]
whine	3	[waɪn]
count	4	[kaʊnt]

4–8. Phonetic Transcription: Stops, Nasals, and Glides With Rhotic Vowels

Phonetically transcribe each word after identifying the number of phonemes in each word.

Word	# of Phonemes	Phonetic Transcription
bird	3	[bɝd]
year	2	[jɪɚ]
bear	2	[bɛɚ]
our	1	[aʊɚ]
core	2	[kɔɚ]
arm	2	[ɑɚm]
tour	2	[tʊɚ]
earn	2	[ɝn]
yarn	3	[jɑɚn]
tire	2	[taɪɚ]
gear	2	[gɪɚ]
cure	3	[kjʊɚ]
war	2	[wɔɚ]
dire	2	[daɪɚ]
more	2	[mɔɚ]

4–9. Phonetic Transcription: Stops, Nasals, and Glides With Rhotic Vowels

Phonetically transcribe each word after identifying the number of phonemes in each word.

Word	# of Phonemes	Phonetic Transcription
term	3	[tɝm]
deer	2	[dɪɚ]
pure	3	[pjɝ]
court	3	[kɔɚt]
yard	3	[jɑɚd]
carp	3	[kɑɚp]
dirt	3	[dɝt]
pear	2	[pɛɚ]
park	3	[pɑɚk]
wire	2	[waɪɚ]
board	3	[bɔɚd]
card	3	[kɑɚd]
hour	1	[aʊɚ]
born	3	[bɔɚn]
wear	2	[wɛɚ]

4–10. Phonetic Transcription: Fricatives, Affricates, and Liquids With Front Vowels

Phonetically transcribe each word after identifying the number of phonemes in each word.

Word	# of Phonemes	Phonetic Transcription
cheese	3	[t͡ʃiz]
fish	3	[fɪʃ]
sledge	4	[slɛd͡ʒ]
sash	3	[sæʃ]
seal	3	[sil]
gel	3	[d͡ʒɛl]
rash	3	[ɹæʃ]
have	3	[hæv]
thief	3	[θif]
sill	3	[sɪl]
ledge	3	[lɛd͡ʒ]
this	3	[ðɪs]
etch	2	[ɛt͡ʃ]
she	2	[ʃi]
wrath	3	[ɹæθ]

4–11. Phonetic Transcription: Fricatives, Affricates, and Liquids With Front Vowels

Phonetically transcribe each word after identifying the number of phonemes in each word.

Word	# of Phonemes	Phonetic Transcription
flash	4	[flæʃ]
is	2	[ɪz]
chief	3	[t͡ʃif]
freeze	4	[fɹiz]
hedge	3	[hɛd͡ʒ]
with	3	[wɪð]
less	3	[lɛs]
jazz	3	[d͡ʒæz]
flesh	4	[flɛʃ]
these	3	[ðiz]
veal	3	[vil]
stitch	4	[stɪt͡ʃ]
says	3	[sɛz]
seize	3	[siz]
hatch	3	[hæt͡ʃ]

4–12. Phonetic Transcription: Fricatives, Affricates, and Liquids With Central and Back Vowels

Phonetically transcribe each word after identifying the number of phonemes in each word.

Word	# of Phonemes	Phonetic Transcription
judge	3	[d͡ʒʌd͡ʒ]
love	3	[lʌv]
shawl	3	[ʃɑl] - [ʃɔl]
the	2	[ðʌ]
full	3	[fʊl]
shoes	3	[ʃuz]
hot	3	[hɑt]
huge	4	[hjud͡ʒ]
chew	2	[t͡ʃu]
jaw	2	[d͡ʒɑ] - [d͡ʒɔ]
fall	3	[fɑl] - [fɔl]
lock	3	[lɑk]
saw	2	[sɑ] - [sɔ]
sludge	4	[slʌd͡ʒ]
rule	3	[ɹul]

4–13. Phonetic Transcription: Fricatives, Affricates, and Liquids With Central and Back Vowels

Phonetically transcribe each word after identifying the number of phonemes in each word.

Word	# of Phonemes	Phonetic Transcription
soothe	3	[suð]
shook	3	[ʃʊk]
fuzz	3	[fʌz]
through	3	[θɹu]
shove	3	[ʃʌv]
choose	3	[t͡ʃuz]
push	3	[pʊʃ]
raw	2	[ɹɑ] - [ɹɔ]
use	3	[juz]
rush	3	[ɹʌʃ]
shot	3	[ʃɑt]
hall	3	[hɑl] - [hɔl]
zoo	2	[zu]
juice	3	[d͡ʒus]
loss	3	[lɑs] - [lɔs]

4–14. Phonetic Transcription: Fricatives, Affricates, and Liquids With Diphthong Vowels

Phonetically transcribe each word after identifying the number of phonemes in each word.

Word	# of Phonemes	Phonetic Transcription
save	3	[seɪv]
loaf	3	[loʊf]
south	3	[saʊθ]
life	3	[laɪf]
soy	2	[sɔɪ]
change	4	[tʃeɪndʒ]
rice	3	[ɹaɪs]
oil	2	[ɔɪl]
those	3	[ðoʊz]
chow	2	[tʃaʊ]
soul	3	[soʊl]
choice	3	[tʃɔɪs]
file	3	[faɪl]
sale	3	[seɪl]
vow	2	[vaʊ]

4–15. Phonetic Transcription: Fricatives, Affricates, and Liquids With Diphthong Vowels

Phonetically transcribe each word after identifying the number of phonemes in each word.

Word	# of Phonemes	Phonetic Transcription
joust	4	[d͡ʒaʊst]
lie	2	[laɪ]
soil	3	[sɔɪl]
chase	3	[t͡ʃeɪs]
hose	3	[hoʊz]
voice	3	[vɔɪs]
jail	3	[d͡ʒeɪl]
sigh	2	[saɪ]
though	2	[ðoʊ]
mouth	3	[maʊθ]
how	2	[haʊ]
joy	2	[d͡ʒɔɪ]
raise	3	[ɹeɪz]
slow	3	[sloʊ]
five	3	[faɪv]

4–16. Phonetic Transcription: Fricatives, Affricates, and Liquids With Rhotic Vowels

Phonetically transcribe each word after identifying the number of phonemes in each word.

Word	# of Phonemes	Phonetic Transcription
lure	2	[luɚ]
fair	2	[f͡ɛɚ]
verse	3	[vɝs]
shore	2	[ʃ͡ɔɚ]
tsar	2	[z͡ɑɚ]
surf	3	[sɝf]
there	2	[ð͡ɛɚ]
veer	2	[v͡ɪɚ]
sour	2	[sa͡ʊɚ]
hair	2	[h͡ɛɚ]
fear	2	[f͡ɪɚ]
church	3	[t͡ʃɝt͡ʃ]
roar	2	[ɹ͡ɔɚ]
higher	2	[ha͡ɪɚ]
sheer	2	[ʃ͡ɪɚ]

4–17. Phonetic Transcription: Fricatives, Affricates, and Liquids With Rhotic Vowels

Phonetically transcribe each word after identifying the number of phonemes in each word.

Word	# of Phonemes	Phonetic Transcription
earth	2	[ɝθ]
sewer	4	[ˈsu.wɚ]
flour	3	[flaʊ͡ɚ]
jar	2	[dʒɑɚ]
cheer	2	[t͡ʃɪɚ]
sore	2	[sɔɚ]
liar	3	[laɪ͡.ɚ]
share	2	[ʃɛɚ]
chore	2	[t͡ʃɔɚ]
chairs	3	[t͡ʃɛɚz]
fire	2	[faɪ͡ɚ]
shower	2	[ʃaʊ͡ɚ]
fur	2	[fɝ]
here	2	[hɪ͡ɚ]
far	2	[fɑ͡ɚ]

4–18. Phonetic Transcription: Disyllabic Words With Front Vowels

Phonetically transcribe each word after identifying the number of phonemes in each word.

Word	# of Phonemes	Phonetic Transcription
vaccine	6	[væk.ˈsin]
taxes	6	[ˈtæk.səz]
eggshell	5	[ˈɛg.ʃɛl]
palate	5	[ˈpæ.lət]
heaven	5	[ˈhɛ.vən]
receipt	5	[ɹə.ˈsit]
basket	6	[ˈbæs.kɪt]
sibling	6	[ˈsɪ.blɪŋ]
discrete	7	[dɪ.ˈskɹit]
lefty	5	[ˈlɛf.ti]
petite	5	[pɪ.ˈtit]
festive	6	[ˈfɛ.stɪv]
prison	6	[ˈpɹɪ.zɪn]
treason	6	[ˈtɹi.zɪn]
fencing	6	[ˈfɛn.sɪŋ]

4–19. Phonetic Transcription: Disyllabic Words With Front Vowels

Phonetically transcribe each word after identifying the number of phonemes in each word.

Word	# of Phonemes	Phonetic Transcription
sheepish	5	[ˈʃi.pɪʃ]
kitten	5	[ˈkɪ.ʔɪn]
magnet	6	[ˈmæg.nət]
caption	6	[ˈkæp.ʃən]
teaches	5	[ˈti.t͡ʃəz]
decrease	6	[di.ˈkɹis]
acting	5	[ˈæk.tɪŋ]
trapeze	6	[tɹæ.ˈpiz]
lesson	5	[ˈlɛ.sən]
wagon	5	[ˈwæ.gən]
helmet	6	[ˈhɛl.mət]
lettuce	5	[ˈlɛ.ɾəs]
gallop	5	[ˈgæ.ləp]
napkin	6	[ˈnæp.kɪn]
zigzag	6	[ˈzɪg.zæg]

4–20. Phonetic Transcription: Disyllabic Words With Central and Back Vowels

Phonetically transcribe each word after identifying the number of phonemes in each word.

Word	# of Phonemes	Phonetic Transcription
jumpy	5	[ˈd͡ʒʌm.pi]
crouton	6	[ˈt͡ʃɑk.lət]
rebuke	6	[ɹə.ˈbjuk]
spoonful	7	[ˈspun.fʊl]
juggle	5	[ˈd͡ʒʌ.gəl]
trouble	6	[ˈtɹʌ.bəl]
cocoon	5	[kə.ˈkun]
also	4	[ˈɑl.so͡ʊ] - [ˈɔl.so͡ʊ]
awful	4	[ˈɑ.fʊl] - [ˈɔ.fʊl]
costume	6	[ˈkɑ.stum]
bubble	5	[ˈbʌ.bəl]
hubris	7	[ˈhju.bɹəs]
stubble	6	[ˈmʌ.ʃɹum]
muscle	5	[ˈmʌ.səl]
unhook	5	[ən.ˈhʊk]

4–21. Phonetic Transcription: Disyllabic Words With Central and Back Vowels

Phonetically transcribe each word after identifying the number of phonemes in each word.

Word	# of Phonemes	Phonetic Transcription
fungus	6	[ˈfʌŋ.gəs]
chocolate	6	[ˈt͡ʃak.lət]
balloon	5	[bə.ˈlun]
quota	5	[ˈkwoʊ͡.ɾə]
jungle	6	[ˈd͡ʒʌŋ.gəl]
glucose	6	[ˈglu.ko͡ʊs]
bottle	5	[ˈbɑ.ɾəl]
oblong	5	[ˈɑ.blɔŋ] - [ˈɑ.blaŋ]
pupil	6	[ˈpju.pəl]
cuckoo	4	[ˈku.ku]
judo	4	[ˈd͡ʒu.do͡ʊ]
bugle	6	[ˈbju.gəl]
mushroom	6	[ˈmʌ.ʃɹum]
couple	5	[ˈkʌ.pəl]
pontoon	6	[pɑn.ˈtun]

4–22. Phonetic Transcription: Disyllabic Words With All Vowels

Phonetically transcribe each word after identifying the number of phonemes in each word.

Word	# of Phonemes	Phonetic Transcription
locket	5	[ˈlɑ.kɪt]
outdo	4	[aʊt.ˈdu]
baboon	5	[bæ.ˈbun]
downy	4	[ˈdaʊ.ni]
renowned	6	[ɹə.ˈnaʊnd]
eyelash	4	[ˈaɪ.læʃ]
input	5	[ˈɪn.pʊt]
storage	5	[ˈstɔɚ.ədʒ]
convoy	5	[ˈkɑn.vɔɪ]
dormant	6	[ˈdɔɚ.mənt]
ozone	4	[ˈoʊ.zoʊn]
chicken	5	[ˈtʃɪ.kɪn]
deter	4	[di.ˈtɚ]
repair	4	[ɹə.ˈpɛɚ]
reading	5	[ˈɹi.ɹɪŋ]

4–23. Phonetic Transcription: Disyllabic Words With All Vowels

Phonetically transcribe each word after identifying the number of phonemes in each word.

Word	# of Phonemes	Phonetic Transcription
chipmunk	7	[ˈt͡ʃɪp.mʌŋk]
safety	5	[ˈseɪf.ti]
message	5	[ˈmɛ.sɪd͡ʒ]
journey	4	[ˈd͡ʒɝ.ni]
mermaid	5	[ˈmɝ.meɪd]
tackle	5	[ˈtæ.kəl]
thoughtful	6	[ˈθɑt.fʊl] - [ˈθɔt.fʊl]
disease	5	[dɪˈziz]
issue	3	[ˈɪ.ʃu]
shovel	5	[ˈʃʌ.vəl]
pulley	4	[ˈpʊ.li]
outlook	5	[ˈaʊt.lʊk]
causeway	5	[kɑz.weɪ]
tarmac	5	[ˈtɑɚ.mæk]
exploit	7	[ɛkˈsplɔɪt]

4–24. Phonetic Transcription: Polysyllabic Words With All Vowels

Phonetically transcribe each word after identifying the number of phonemes in each word.

Word	# of Phonemes	Phonetic Transcription
recycle	7	[ɹi.ˈsaɪ.kəl]
firemen	5	[ˈfaɪɚ.mɛn]
ponytail	7	[ˈpoʊ.ni.teɪl]
triangle	8	[ˈtɹaɪ.æŋ.gəl]
application	9	[æ.plɪ.ˈkeɪ.ʃən]
advantage	8	[æd.ˈvæn.tɪdʒ]
amplifier	7	[ˈæm.plə.faɪɚ]
knowingly	6	[ˈnoʊ.ɪŋ.li]
judgment	7	[ˈdʒʌdʒ.mɛnt]
enlighten	7	[ɛn.ˈlaɪ.tən]
holiday	6	[ˈhɑ.lə.deɪ]
beginning	7	[bə.ˈgɪ.nɪŋ]
tableware	7	[ˈteɪ.bəl.wɛɚ]
unicorn	7	[ˈju.nə.kɔɚn]
piggy bank	8	[ˈpɪ.gi.bæŋk]

4–25. Phonetic Transcription: Polysyllabic Words With All Vowels

Phonetically transcribe each word after identifying the number of phonemes in each word.

Word	# of Phonemes	Phonetic Transcription
rectangle	9	[ˈɹɛk.tæŋ.gəl]
president	9	[ˈpɹɛ.zɪ.ɾənt]
language	7	[ˈlæŋ.gwɪd͡ʒ]
ordinary	6	[ˈɔɚ.ɾɪ.nɛɚ.i]
exchange	7	[ɛks.ˈt͡ʃeɪnd͡ʒ]
disqualify	10	[dɪ.ˈskwɑ.lɪ.faɪ]
confidence	10	[ˈkɑn.fɪ.dɪnts]
thousand	6	[ˈθaʊ.zənd]
minority	7	[maɪ.ˈnɔɚ.ɪ.ɾi]
buoyant	6	[ˈbɔɪ.jənt]
zucchini	6	[zu.ˈki.ni]
everything	7	[ˈɛv.ɹi.θɪŋ]
quintuplet	10	[kwɪn.ˈtʌ.plət]
Blackbeard	7	[blæk.bɪɚd]
themselves	8	[ðɛm.ˈsɛlvz]

4–26. Phonetic Transcription: Polysyllabic Words With All Vowels

Phonetically transcribe each word after identifying the number of phonemes in each word.

Word	# of Phonemes	Phonetic Transcription
childhood	7	['tʃaɪld.hʊd]
bullying	6	['bʊ.li.ɪŋ]
coordinate	8	[koʊ.'ɔɚ.ɾɪ.neɪt']
annual	6	['æn.ju.ʊl]
relaxation	10	[ɹi.læk.'seɪ.ʃən]
invisible	9	[ɪn.'vɪ.zɪ.bəl]
adversity	8	[æd.'vɝ.sɪ.ɾi]
forgiveness	8	[fɔɚ.'gɪv.nəs]
insomniac	9	[ɪn.'sɑm.ni.æk]
captivate	8	[kæp.tɪ.veɪt]
ignition	7	[ɪg.'nɪ.ʃən]
jellyfish	7	['dʒɛ.li.fɪʃ]
obesity	7	[oʊ.'bi.sɪ.ɾi]
Thursday	5	['θɝz.deɪ]
exhaling	8	[ɛks.'heɪ.lɪŋ]

4–27. Phonetic Transcription: Same-Vowel Phrases

Phonetically transcribe each phrase.

Phrase	Phonetic Transcription
flea sneezed	[fli snizd]
shrimp primped	[ʃɹɪmp pɹɪmpt]
whale ailed	[weɪl eɪld]
hen bent	[hɛn bɛnt]
cat sat	[kæt sæt]
bug hugged	[bʌg hʌgd]
bird heard	[bɝd hɝd]
moose mused	[mus mjuzd]
wolf put	[wʊlf pʊt]
roach joked	[ɹoʊtʃ dʒoʊkt]
hog brawled	[hɑg bɹɑld] - [hɔg bɹɔld]
fox trotted	[fɑks ˈtɹɑ.ɹɪd]
fly sighed	[flaɪ saɪd]
chow-chow bowed	[tʃaʊ tʃaʊ baʊd]
koi destroyed	[kɔɪ dɛ.ˈstɹɔɪd]

4–28. Reading Phonetic Transcription: Same-Vowel Phrases

Orthographically write each phonetically transcribed phrase. Remember that there are no capital phonetic symbols.

Phonetic Transcription	Phrase
[li bimz]	Lee/Li beams.
[d͡ʒɪl bɪldz]	Jill builds.
[d͡ʒeɪd eɪks]	Jade aches.
[bɛl bɛts]	Belle bets.
[æn ækts]	Ann acts.
[t͡ʃʌk wʌn]	Chuck won.
[pɝl wɝlz]	Pearl whirls.
[kɹuz t͡ʃuz]	Cruz chews.
['wʊ.di lʊks]	Woody looks.
[bo͡ʊ d͡ʒo͡ʊks]	Beau jokes.
[pɑl nɑz] - [pɔl nɔz]	Paul gnaws.
[tɑʒ dɹɑps]	Taj drops.
[ma͡ɪ kɹa͡ɪz]	Mai cries.
[kla͡ʊs ha͡ʊlz]	Klaus howls.
[ɹɔ͡ɪ d͡ʒɔ͡ɪnz]	Roy joins.

4–29. Reading Phonetic Transcription: Front Vowels With Different Spellings

Orthographically write each phonetically transcribed word.

Phonetic Transcription	Word
[ni]	knee
[ki]	key
[mi]	me
[si]	sea see
[snɪf]	sniff
['wɪ.mɪn] - ['wɪ.mən]	women
[θɹɛd]	thread
[sɛd]	said
[bɛd]	bed
[kæt͡ʃ]	catch
[kæn]	can

4–30. Reading Phonetic Transcription: Central and Back Vowels With Different Spellings

Orthographically write each phonetically transcribed word.

Phonetic Transcription	Word
[lʌʃ]	lush
[dʌn]	done
[blɑg] - [blɔg]	blog
[hɑt] - [hɔt]	hot
[mun]	moon
[tun]	tune
[hʊd]	hood
[ʃʊd]	should
[ɑt] - [ɔt]	ought
[kɑt] - [kɔt]	caught

4–31. Reading Phonetic Transcription: Diphthongs With Different Spellings

Orthographically write each phonetically transcribed word.

Phonetic Transcription	Word
[ta͡ɪ]	tie
[sa͡ɪ]	sigh
[fla͡ɪ]	fly
[ha͡ɪ]	hi
[ha͡ɪst̚]	heist
[ba͡ɪt]	bite
[ba͡ʊ.wa͡ʊ]	bow-wow
[pla͡ʊd]	ploughed
[bɔ͡ɪz]	boys
[nɔ͡ɪz]	noise
[ɹe͡ɪ]	ray
[we͡ɪ]	weigh
[we͡ɪst]	waste
[we͡ɪt]	wait
[ko͡ʊm]	comb
[ho͡ʊm]	home

4–32. Diacritical Marks for Consonants

1. Match each state of the glottis with its corresponding diacritical mark.

   voiceless   __c__   a. [x̱]

   aspirated   __b__   b. [xʰ]

   voiced   __d__   c. [x̥]

   creaky   __a__   d. [x̰]

2. Narrowly transcribe each of the following words using the appropriate diacritical mark.

   a. *teeth* produced with tongue tip touching the back of the upper   [t̪iθ]
   incisors for /t/

   b. *zoo* produced with blade of the tongue used to produce [z]   [z̻u]

   c. *one* produced with a nasalized word-initial consonant   [w̃ʌn]

   d. *zip* produced by lateralizing [z]   [zˡɪp]

   e. *tap* produced by unreleasing the word-final stop phoneme   [tæp̚]

   f. *juice* produced by prolonging the final consonant   [d͡ʒusː]

   g. *bottle* produced with a syllabic final consonantt   ['bɑd.l̩]

4–33. Marking Primary Stress in Disyllabic Words

Include the primary stress diacritic in your phonetic transcription of each of the following prepositions.

1. beside   [bi.'saɪd]

2. anti   ['æn.taɪ]

3. during   ['dɝ.ɪŋ]

4. within   [wɪ.'ðɪn]

5. versus   ['vɝ.sɪs]

6. into   ['ɪn.tu]

7. beyond   [bi.'jand]

8. inside   [ɪn.'saɪd]

9. onto   ['an.tu] - ['ɔn.tu]

10. without   [wɪ.'ðaʊt]

4–34. Using the Tap Allophone

Circle "yes" or "no" to indicate whether the /t/ or /d/ phoneme can be replaced by a tap. Then phonetically transcribe each word, using the tap allophone where possible. If the tap cannot be used, briefly explain why.

1. letter   **yes** / no   ['lɛ.ɾɚ]

2. watt   yes / **no**   [wɑt]   No, because **tt is not between two vowel sounds.**

3. cattail   yes / **no**   ['kæt:.e͡ɪl]   No, because **both t sounds are pronounced.**

4. cigarette   yes / **no**   [sɪ.gə.'ɹɛt]   No, because **"tt" is followed by a silent e.**

5. little   **yes** / no   ['lɪ.ɾəl]

6. ditto   **yes** / no   ['dɪ.ɾo͡ʊ]

7. attack   yes / **no**   [ə.'tæk]   No, because **second syllable is stressed.**

8. attic   **yes** / no   ['æ.ɾɪk]

9. attention   yes / **no**   [ə'tɛn.ʃən]   No, because **second syllable with "t" is stressed.**

10. odd   yes / **no**   [ɑd]   No, because **"dd" is not between two vowels.**

11. adding   **yes** / no   ['æ.ɾɪŋ]

12. addition   yes / **no**   [ə.'dɪ.ʃən]   No, because **second syllable with "d" is stressed.**

13. cheddar   **yes** / no   ['t͡ʃɛ.ɾɚ]

14. buddy   **yes** / no   ['bʌ.ɾi]

15. ado   yes / **no**   [ə'du]   No, because **second syllable with "d" is stressed.**

SUPRASEGMENTAL FEATURES OF SPEECH

5–1. Stress: Identifying and Diagramming Stress in Words

Underline the stressed syllables in each pair of words. Then diagram the stress pattern. An example has been done for you.

Example:

    instant   inform

    ———   ———

        ———   ———

    in   stant   in   **form**

1. unless   under

        ———   ———

    ———   ———

    un   **less**   **un**   der

2. effect   affect

        ———   ———

    ———   ———

    e   **ffect**   **a**   ffect

3. supper   support

    ———   ———

        ———   ———

    su   pper   su   **pport**

4. between   beacon

———   ———

———   ———

be   **tween**   **bea**   con

5. beckon   because

———   ———

———   ———

be   ckon   be   **cause**

6. about   able

———   ———

———   ———

ɑ   **bout**   **ɑ**   ble

7. away   awesome

———   ———

———   ———

ɑ   **way**   **awe**   some

8. disagree   disaggregate

———   ———

———   ———   ———   ———   ———   ———   ———

dis   ɑ   **gree**   dis   **ɑ**   **g**gre   gate

9. against   agency

———   ———

———   ———   ———

ɑ   **gainst**   **ɑ**   gen   cy

10. acre   across

———   ———   ———

———   ———

ɑ   cre   ɑ   **cross**

11. agate   again

_____   _____

      _____   _____

a   gate   a   **gain**

12. around   Arabic

      _____   _____

_____   _____ _____

a   **round**   **Ar**   a   bic

13. between   Beatrice

      _____   _____

_____   _____ _____

be   **tween**   **Be**   a   trice

14. Beckman   because

_____   _____

      _____   _____

Beck man   be   **cause**

15. canopy   control

_____   _____

      _____ _____   _____

ca   no   py   con   **trol**

16. create   crease

      _____   _____

_____

cre   **ate**   **crease**

17. himself   hymnal

      _____   _____

_____   _____

him   **self**   **hym** nal

18. pumice   police

    _____   _____

       _____   _____

    pu   mice   po   **lice**

19. until   unanimous

       _____   _____

    _____   _____   _____

    un   **til**   u   **na**   ni   mous

20. wither   within

    _____   _____

       _____   _____

    wi   ther   with   **in**

21. witness   without

    _____   _____

       _____   _____

    wit   ness   with   **out**

22. polar   polite

    _____   _____

       _____   _____

    po   lar   po   **lite**

5–2. Stress: Identifying Stress in Different Forms of the Same Word

Underline the stressed syllables in the following words.

  1. interpret   interpreter   interpretation

  2. wonder   wonderful   wonderfully

  3. remain   remainder   remaining

  4. icon   iconic   iconicity

  5. agree   agreement   agreeable

  6. apply   applicant   application

7. <u>ad</u>vertise   <u>ad</u>vertising   adver<u>tise</u>ment

8. be<u>lieve</u>   be<u>liev</u>able   believa<u>bil</u>ity

9. i<u>deal</u>   i<u>deal</u>ize   i<u>dea</u>lly

10. <u>na</u>vigate   <u>na</u>vigator   navi<u>ga</u>tion

11. <u>le</u>mon   <u>le</u>monade

12. <u>king</u>   <u>king</u>dom

5–3. Syntactic Phrases: Saying One Utterance Using Two Different Phrase Units

Produce each utterance using two different phrase units.

1. Let's cook grandpa dinner tonight.

    Let's cook grandpa dinner tonight.

    Let's cook, grandpa; dinner tonight?

2. I saw a man eating chicken.

    I saw a man, eating chicken.

    I saw a man-eating chicken.

3. Twenty five dollar bills.

    Twenty five-dollar bills.

    Twenty-five dollar bills

4. It's raining children.

    It's raining, children.

    It's raining children!

5. I'm sorry I love you.

    I'm sorry I love you.

    I'm sorry. I love you!

6. I find joy in cooking my family and my dog.

    I find joy in cooking my family and my dog!

    I find joy in cooking, my family, and my dog.

5–4. Intonation: Saying Sentences With Specified Intonation Contours

Practice saying each utterance using the intonation contour diagrammed.

1. I saw you yesterday.

2. I saw you yesterday?

3. She likes burgers and fries.

4. Did your brother text you?

5. What time will you be ready?

5–5. Intonation: Saying Sentences With Specified Intonation Contours

Write an utterance that could fit each intonation contour diagrammed.

1. <u>Answers will vary.</u>

2.

3.

4.

5.

5–6. Prosody: Saying One Utterance Using Two Different Phrase Units

Practice saying each of the following nonsense phrases until you come up with a commonly used term.

1.	foe net ick sigh ants	**phonetic science**
2.	overt a reign bow	**over the rainbow**
3.	are tick you lay shun	**articulation**
4.	poor to Lynn door a gun	**Portland, Oregon**
5.	bolt Tim more merry Lynn	**Baltimore, Maryland**
6.	cam bow Dee ha	**Cambodia**
7.	wall diss knee	**Walt Disney**
8.	hair reap otter	**Harry Potter**
9.	jewel yeehaw rob hurts	**Julia Roberts**
10.	chess ape eek bay	**Chesapeake Bay**
11.	wheel ute ants we the me	**Will you dance with me?**
12.	kid tea vee dee oh	**kitty video**

6

ACOUSTIC PHONETICS

6–1. Acoustic Terms

1. A wave resulting from an up and down movement wave that travels side to side is a **transverse** wave.

2. If a movement and the resulting pressure wave travel in the same direction the wave is **longitudinal**.

3. Sound waves are which type of wave? **longitudinal**.

4. When molecules are farther apart from each than they are in their resting position, it is called **rarefaction**.

5. Molecules that are closer together than they are in their resting position are in a state called **compression**.

6. Air pressure variations over time can be graphed on a **waveform**.

7. Decibels measure **intensity** / frequency.

8. Hertz measure intensity / **frequency**.

6–2. Acoustic Phonetic Terms

1. Frequency is the objective representation of **pitch**.

2. Loudness is a subjective representation of **intensity**.

3. How are frequency and time related?
   Frequency is defined as the number of cycles or repetitions that a sound wave completes in a period of time. Frequency is indicated in hertz (Hz). For example, sound can travel at a frequency of 150 cycles per second = 150 Hz.

4. Define fundamental frequency.
   In speech, fundamental frequency (F0) is related to the number of times the vocal folds vibrate per second. It is an objective measurement.

5. What fundamental frequency differences are observed between biological males and biological females? What differences in fundamental frequency are observed between adults and children?

Typically, biological male voices are associated with a lower F0, and biological female voices are associated with a higher F0. Children have a higher F0 as compared to adults.

6–3. Waveforms

1. Is the following waveform periodic or aperiodic? How can you tell?

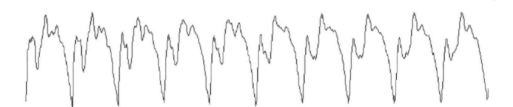

It is periodic. You can tell because it has a repeating pattern.

2. Which of the following waveforms shows a pure tone? Which of the following shows speech?

A.

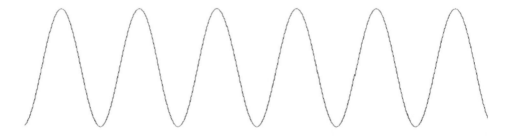

B.

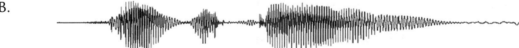

Waveform in A is a pure tone.

Waveform in B is of speech.

6–4. Calculating Fundamental Frequency

1. The duration of the following Waveform A is 0.044 s. Calculate F0:

Waveform A

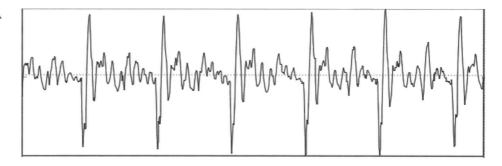

Waveform A is approximately 6.25 cycles/0.044 s.
F0 of ~142 Hz

2. The duration of the following Waveform B is .029 s. Calculate F0:

Waveform B

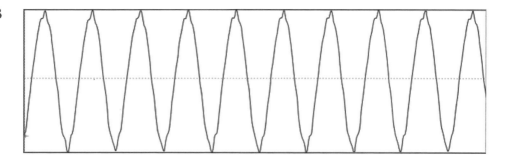

Waveform B is approximately 9.6 cycles/0.029 s.
F0 of ~331 Hz

3. The duration of the following Waveform C is .038 s. Calculate F0:

Waveform C

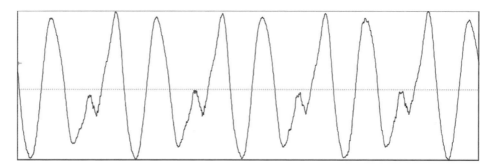

Waveform C is approximately 4.5 cycles/.038 s.
F0 of ~118 Hz

4. Which of the previous waveforms has the highest F0? The lowest F0?

Waveform B has the highest F0 at 331 Hz. It would be perceived as the highest pitch.

Waveform C has the lowest F0 at 118 Hz. It would be perceived as the lowest pitch.

6–5. Waveform Word Matching

1. Match the waveforms to the five words that follow. How did you make each decision?

stop   beep   four   aim   witch

A.

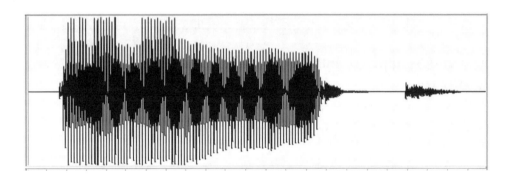

Waveform A is of the word **beep** [bip].

Waveform A is a periodic wave, followed by silence, then a sharp burst of sound and aperiodicity at the end. The change in amplitude for the voiced portion of the wave suggests a voiced consonant followed by a vowel. The burst suggests a voiceless obstruent at the end of the word.

B.

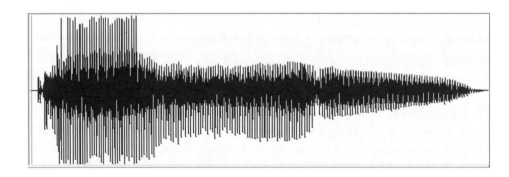

Waveform B is of the word **aim** [eɪm].

Waveform B is a periodic wave throughout with higher intensity at the beginning and a decrease in intensity in the second portion, which fits with a diphthong onset where the dynamic movement is from low to high position. There is a brief but sharp decrease in intensity, suggesting articulatory closure, followed by an increase and gradual decrease in intensity, suggesting a voiced sonorant consonant.

C.

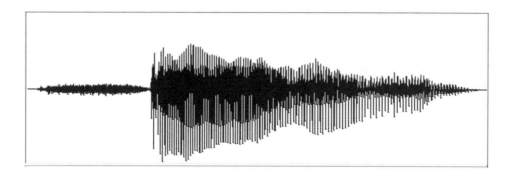

Waveform C is of the word *four* [fɔɚ].

Waveform C begins with an aperiodic sound of low intensity. There is no sharp onset, thereby suggesting a fricative. This segment is followed by a periodic wave that is more intense at the onset suggesting a dipthong vowel.

D.

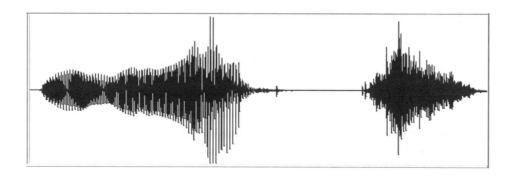

Waveform D is of the word *witch* [wɪtʃ].

Waveform D is periodic at onset, increasing in intensity as it transitions to another periodic portion, suggesting a sonorant followed by a vowel. The word ends with silence followed by an aperiodic sound, suggesting a voiceless affricate.

E.

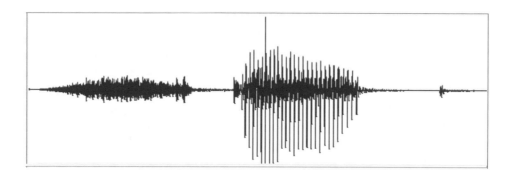

Waveform E is of the word *stop* [stɑp].

Waveform E starts with aperiodicity and low intensity, followed by a period of very low intensity. These two portions suggest a fricative followed by a voiceless unaspirated stop. This is followed by high intensity periodicity, suggesting a vowel. The last portion is silence followed by a weak period of intensity, suggesting another voiceless stop.

6–6. Spectrogram Definitions

1. On a spectrogram, what is the relationship between F1 and tongue height? F2 and tongue advancement?

    F1 and tongue height have an inverse relationship. The higher the vowel, the lower F1 will be.

    F2 and tongue advancement are related in that the more forward the tongue is, the higher F2 will be.

2. For the following vowels, describe the expected F1 and F2 based on tongue placement.

    [u]: **Produced with the tongue high and back so F1 (height) will be low and F2 (advancement) will be low.**

    [i]: **Produced with the tongue high and front so F1 will be low and F2 will be high.**

    [æ]: **Produced with the tongue low and front so F1 will be high and F2 will be high (but since slightly further back in the mouth, not as high as [i]).**

    [ɑ]: **Produced with the tongue low and back so F1 will be high and F2 will be low.**

    [aɪ]: **Because [aɪ] is a diphthong, the formants will transition from [a] to [ɪ]. [a] is a low central vowel so F1 will be high and F2 will be mid. [ɪ] is a high front vowel so F1 will be low and F2 will be high.**

6–7. Articulatory Versus Acoustic Space for Vowels

1. On the following grid, plot the vowels in the acoustic space. Each tick mark on the grid is 100 Hz.

   Vowel 1. F1: 280 F2: 2300

   Vowel 2. F1: 700 F2: 2000

   Vowel 3. F1: 640 F2: 1250

   Vowel 4. F1: 320 F2: 1300

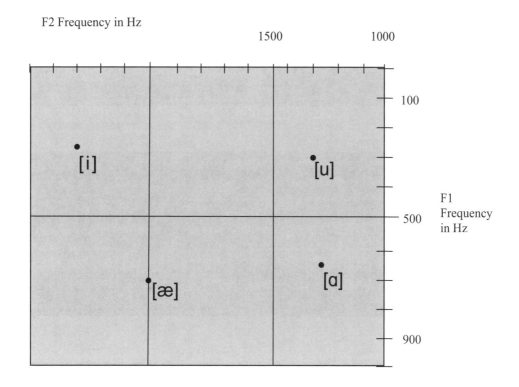

2. Identify these four vowel phonemes based on their position in the acoustic space.

   a. Vowel 1: [i]

   b. Vowel 2: [æ]

   c. Vowel 3: [ɑ]

   d. Vowel 4: [u]

6–8. Spectrogram Vowel Matching

Match the following spectrograms with the monophthong or diphthong vowels. Explain the acoustic features that were used to match the vowel to the spectrogram.

[ɔɪ]   [ɪ]   [ɑ]   [aʊ]   [u]

A.

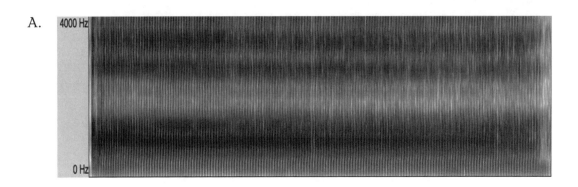

B.

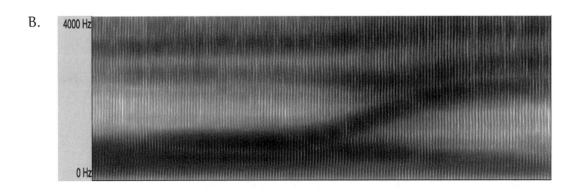

C.

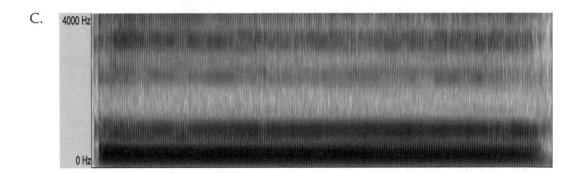

D.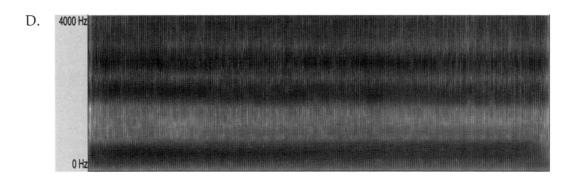

E.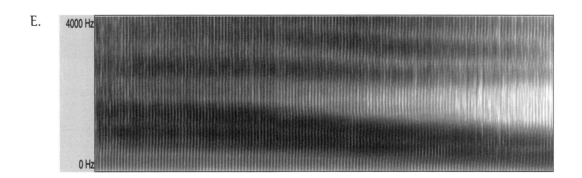

a. [ɑ] F1 and F2 are very close together and are both low frequency. F1 is just below and F2 is just above 1000 Hz. While F3 and F4 are clear in this spectrogram, we do not need to measure them to determine the vowel phoneme.

b. [ɔɪ] There is a clear transition in both F1 and F2 formants, suggesting a dipthong that changes in tongue height and tongue advancement. The F1 transition is slight, from approximately 450 Hz to 350 Hz, suggesting a slight increase in vowel height. The F1 suggests that the vowel started at mid tongue height. The F2 transition is greater, shifting from approximately 800 Hz to 2100 Hz, indicating that the tongue has moved forward in the mouth.

c. [u] The vowel formants do not change frequency, which indicates the vowel is a monophthong. There is a small gap between F1 and F2. There is a very low F1, measured at ~400 Hz in the middle of the formant band. F2 is distinct from F1 with a midpoint frequency of ~1000 Hz.

d. [ɪ] Steady-state vowel. F1 is low, at approximately 400 Hz, suggesting a high vowel. F2 is higher at about 2000 Hz, suggesting a front vowel. There is a significant gap between F1 and F2.

e. [aʊ] F1 and F2 both decrease in frequency, suggesting a diphthong. The tongue shifts from a low to a high position (since F1 decreases) and retracts during the latter portion of the diphthong, moving slightly further back in the mouth (since F2 decreases slightly).

6–9. Matching Spectrograms

Spectrograms A through F are of [ʌ.Cʌ] productions, the [C] representing a consonant phoneme of English. Each spectrogram shows acoustic energy from 0 to 4000 Hz. Match the following consonant phonemes to their spectrogram, briefly describing how you found your answer.

[m]   [k]   [s]   [d͡ʒ]   [ʃ]   [ɹ]

A.

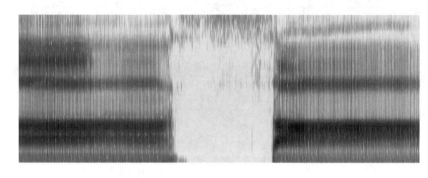

B.

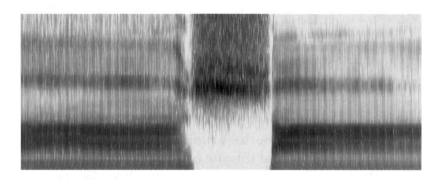

C.

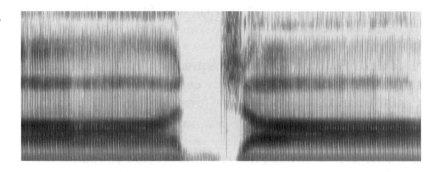

D.

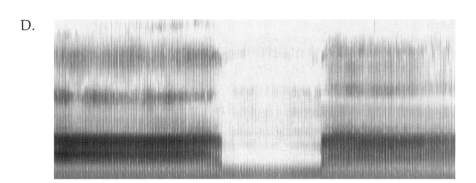

E.

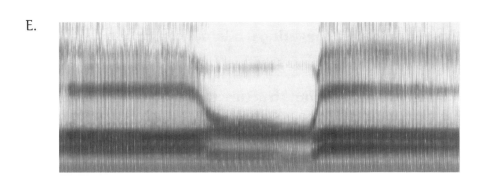

F.

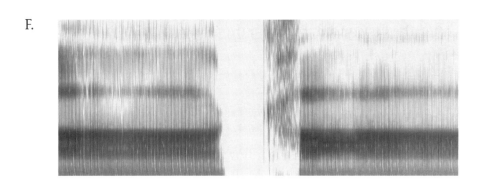

Spectrogram A: [s]

The disturbance pattern is typical of voiceless fricatives. The disturbance is high frequency (most of it above 4000 Hz, which you can't see). We know it is voiceless because there are random aperiodic striations throughout the consonant.

Spectrogram B: [ʃ]

The disturbance pattern is typical of voiceless fricatives. The disturbance starts at a lower frequency than Spectrogram A, which is also a fricative. There is no voicing present and there are random aperiodic striations throughout the consonant.

Spectrogram C: [d͡ʒ]

This spectrogram shows a sharp end to the initial vowel, suggesting a stop closure. There are periodic vibrations during the stop closure, suggesting it is voiced. There are aperiodic striations after the stop closure, suggesting frication. It looks like a combination of a stop and the fricative [ʃ], which implies an English affricate. Due to the voicing seen before the release, it can be determined to be the voiced affricate [d͡ʒ].

Spectrogram D: [m]

The key component of Spectrogram D is the faint formant structure throughout the consonant, which is typical of nasals. There is a weak nasal bar at low frequency, also typical for nasal phonemes. Before and after the consonant, F1 and F2 drop slightly, which is indicative of lip closure, suggesting a bilabial consonant.

Spectrogram E: [ɹ]

In spectrogram E, there is clear formant structure throughout the consonant, which is typical of voiced approximants. F3 drops significantly, which is a hallmark characteristic of the rhotic [ɹ].

Spectrogram F: [k]

The closure and sudden release is typically seen in stops. Due to the silence before the burst and the visible aspiration after the release, the stop is voiceless. F2 and F3 join both before and after the consonant, forming the "velar pinch," indicating velar place of articulation.

6–10. Segmenting Waveforms

The following six words are represented in the following spectrograms—spectrogram A, B, and C. There are two words in each spectrogram. Match each word to its corresponding spectrogram. Below each spectrogram, transcribe each word and segment each spectrogram.

doom   ballistic   statistic   mines   mood   prince

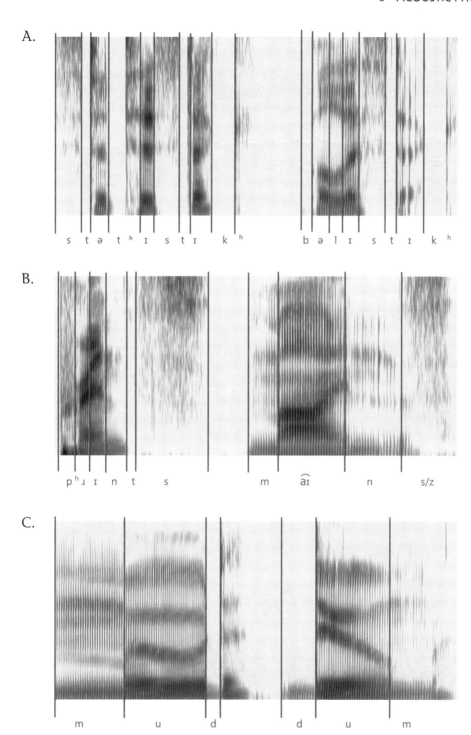

Spectrogram A: *statistic*   *ballistic*

Spectrogram B: *prints*   *mines*

Spectrogram C: *mood*   *doom*

6–11. Spectrogram Sentence Reading

Match each of the following spectrograms—labeled A, B, and C—with one of the following phrases. There are extra phrases provided to increase the challenge.

Run really fast.

It's time.

The dog is outside.

Hang on to my ring.

Please stop and think.

What is the answer to the question?

A.
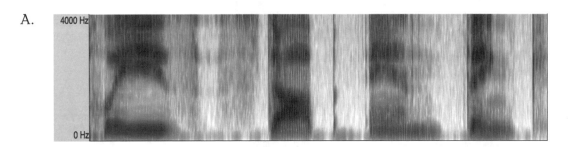

B.
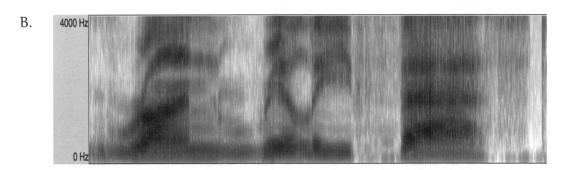

C.
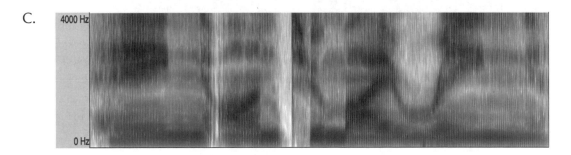

Spectrogram A: ***Please stop and think.***

Spectrogram B: ***Run really fast.***

Spectrogram C: ***Hang on to my ring.***

6–12. Try It Yourself: Wavesurfer and Praat Download Links

Try making your own waveforms and spectrograms with the free downloadable software, Wavesurfer or Praat! You can explore different user interfaces and capabilities using these software.

Free Praat download for Windows:
http://www.fon.hum.uva.nl/praat/download_win.html

Free Praat download for Mac:
http://www.fon.hum.uva.nl/praat/download_mac.html

Free Wavesurfer download at https://sourceforge.net/projects/wavesurfer/

CONSONANT PHONOLOGY

7–1. Syllabicity: Identifying Parts of Syllables

Fill in the missing information.

Orthographic Transcription	Phonetic Transcription	Onset	Rime	Nucleus	Coda
send	sɛnd	s	ɛnd	ɛ	nd
tries	tɹaɪz	tɹ	aɪz	aɪ	z
mist	mɪst	m	ɪst	ɪ	st
act	ækt		ækt	æ	kt
bee	bi	b	i	i	
play	pleɪ	pl	eɪ	eɪ	
crooks	kɹʊks	kɹ	ʊks	ʊ	ks
lunch	lʌntʃ	l	ʌntʃ	ʌ	ntʃ

7–2. Stops: Identifying Words With Syllable-Initial Aspiration

Circle the words for which the syllable-initial stop aspiration rule could apply.

taxi	stay	**carrot**	baggage
paper	letter	**apple**	**cook**
baton	native	**king**	speak
kick	winner	**two**	novice
money	**target**	**park**	slate
upon	music	skill	**economy**
rain	witch	fake	**support**

7–3. Stops: Identifying and Transcribing Words With Syllable-Initial Aspiration

Circle the word in each pair for which the syllable-initial stop aspiration rule could apply. Then transcribe each word.

Word A	Word B	Transcription A	Transcription B
squid	**kid**	skwɪd	kʰɪd
atop	stop	ə.ˈtʰɑp	stɑp
bobbing	**popping**	ˈbɑ.bɪŋ	pʰɑ.pɪŋ
stark	**tarp**	stɑɚ͡k	tʰɑɚ͡p
toggle	boggle	ˈtʰɑ.ɡəl	ˈbɑ.ɡəl
carry	scary	ˈkʰɛɚ͡.i	ˈskɛɚ͡.i
spot	**pot**	spɑt	pʰɑt
bye	**pie**	ba͡ɪ	pʰa͡ɪ

7–4. Stops: Identifying Words With Word-Final Unreleased Stops

Circle the words for which the word-final unreleased stop rule could apply.

ship	**back**	dome	**top**
fire	**mat**	doctor	chalet
rot	cheese	**pick**	loss
lamb	farm	**can't**	**salt**
rope	patch	myth	**map**
complete	swirl	buzz	**attack**

7–5. Stops: Identifying and Transcribing Words With Word-Final Unreleased Stops

Circle the word in each pair for which the word-final unreleased stop rule could apply. Then transcribe each word.

Word A	Word B	Transcription A	Transcription B
can't	band	kænt˺	bænd
shrug	**shuck**	ʃɹʌg	ʃʌk˺
hip	glib	hɪp˺	glɪb
grand	**art**	gɹænd	a͡ɚt˺
teacup	bathtub	ˈti.kəp˺	ˈbæθ.təb
walled	**wallet**	wɑld	ˈwɑ.lət˺
bullfrog	**garlic**	ˈbʊl.fɹɑg	ˈga͡ɚ.lɪk˺
plate	played	ple͡ɪt˺	ple͡ɪd
loop	lobe	lup˺	lo͡ʊb
bag	**back**	bæg	bæk˺
knit	node	nɪt˺	no͡ʊd
snip	crib	snɪp˺	kɹɪb

7–6. Stops: Identifying Words With Unreleased Stops in Stop + Stop Clusters or When Preceding Syllabic Nasals

1. Circle the words for which the unreleased stop in a stop + stop cluster rule could apply.

wagged	**whipped**	**trucked**	dictate
inducted	**baked**	haste	**hoped**
bacteria	octopus	bracelet	fiction
teacher	doctor	lawyer	engineer

2. Circle the words for which the unreleased stop preceding a syllabic nasal rule could apply.

kitten	fasten	fashion	**lighten**
atom	**fatten**	**satin**	settle
mission	kitchen	**leaden**	**batten**
sadden	**bottom**	lentil	even

7–7. Stops: Identifying Words With Unaspirated Stops in /s/ + Stop Clusters

Circle the words for which the unaspirated stop in /s/ + stop cluster rule could apply.

scene	**spill**	**sky**	**stop**
style	**scam**	psychology	**mister**
fasten	**skip**	**scale**	**speckle**
slap	scent	**spam**	scythe
whisker	swan	**school**	**square**
rescue	**chopstick**	sweater	**spatula**
haystack	**snowstorm**	**teaspoon**	**basket**

7–8. Stops: Identifying and Transcribing Words With Unaspirated Stops in /s/ + Stop Clusters

Circle the word in each pair for which the unaspirated stop in /s/ + stop clusters rule could apply. Then transcribe each word.

Word A	Word B	Transcription A	Transcription B
scale	kale	sk͈͡eɪl	kʰe͡ɪl
sunk	**skunk**	sʌŋk	sk͈ʌŋk
slid	**skid**	slɪd	sk͈ɪd
smile	**style**	sma͡ɪl	st͈a͡ɪl
smoke	**spoke**	smo͡ʊk	sp͈o͡ʊk
costume	consume	ˈkas.t͈um	ˈkən.sum
telescope	telephone	ˈtɛ.lə.sk͈o͡ʊp	ˈtɛ.lə.fo͡ʊn
snow	**storm**	sno͡ʊ	st͈ɔ͡˞m
banister	banish	ˈbæ.nɪ.st͈˞	ˈbæ.nɪʃ
sting	swing	st͈ɪŋ	swɪŋ
busy bee	**biscuit**	ˈbɪ.zi ˈbi	ˈbɪ.sk͈ɪt
apostrophe	apology	ə.ˈpa.st͈ɹə.fi	ə.ˈpa.lə.d͡ʒi

7–9. Stops: Identifying and Transcribing Words With Labialized Stops

Circle the words for which the labialized rule could apply to the stop preceding the vowel. Then transcribe each word.

Word	Transcription
poke	pʷo͡ʊk
beat	bit
took	tʷʊk
dime	da͡ɪm
quick	kʷwɪk
goose	gʷus
pop	pɑp
boot	bʷut
take	te͡ɪk
dome	dʷo͡ʊm
squirt	skʷwɝt
good	gʷʊd

7–10. Stops: Identifying and Transcribing Words With Dentalized Alveolar Stops

Circle the words for which the dentalized rule could apply to the alveolar stop preceding /θ/. Then transcribe each word.

Word	Transcription
length	lɛŋkθ
width	wɪd̪θ
breadth	bɹɛd̪θ
depth	dɛpθ
bandwidth	ˈbæn.dwɪd̪θ
hundredth	ˈhʌn.dɹɛd̪θ
birthday	ˈbɝθ.de͡ɪ
mythical	ˈmɪ.θə.kəl
thousandth	ˈθa͡ʊ.zənd̪θ
eighth	e͡ɪt̪θ

7–11. Stops: Identifying and Transcribing Words With Advanced Velar Stops

Circle the words for which the advanced velar stop rule could apply. Then transcribe each word.

Word	Transcription
keep	k̟ip
kept	k̟ɛpt
cop	kɑp
cape	k̟e͡ɪp
ghost	go͡ʊst
give	g̟ɪv
get	g̟ɛt
goose	gus
weak	wik̟
woke	wo͡ʊk
stick	stɪk̟
sag	sæg̟

7–12. Stops: Identifying and Transcribing Words With Glottal Replacements

Circle the word in each pair for which the alveolar stop preceding a syllabic /n/ is replaced with a glottal stop rule could apply. Then transcribe each word.

Word A	Word B	Transcription A	Transcription B
kitten	bottom	ˈkɪ.ʔn̩	ˈbɑ.ɾəm
leaden	sweater	ˈlɛ.ʔn̩	ˈswɛ.ɾɚ
written	tomato	ˈɹɪ.ʔn̩	tə.ˈmeɪ.ɾoʊ
doctor	**fightin'**	ˈdɑk.tɚ	ˈfaɪ.ʔn̩
Sweden	sweeter	ˈswi.ʔn̩	ˈswi.ɾɚ
baton	**rotten**	bə.ˈtɑn	ˈɹɑ.ʔn̩
sagging	**satin**	ˈsæ.ɡɪŋ	ˈsæ.ʔn̩
heighten	butter	ˈhaɪ.ʔn̩	ˈbʌ.ɾɚ
battery	**button**	ˈbæ.ɾɚ.i	ˈbʌ.ʔn̩

7–13. Stops: Identifying and Transcribing Words With Nasal Releases

Circle the words for which the stop preceding a syllabic nasal is released with nasal plosion rule could apply. Then transcribe each word.

Word	Transcription
sadden	ˈsæ.d^{n}n̩
shouldn't	ˈʃʊ.d^{n}n̩t
vacuum	ˈvæ.kjum
happen	ˈhæ.p^{n}n̩
become	bə.ˈkʌm
couldn't	ˈkʊ.d^{n}n̩t
ignite	ɪg.ˈna͡ɪt
upon	ə.ˈpɑn
burden	ˈbɝ.d^{n}n̩
administer	æd.ˈmɪn.ə.stɚ
succumb	sə.ˈkʌm
mannequin	ˈmæ.nə.k^{n}n̩

7–14. Stops: Transcribing Words With Lateral Releases

Circle the correct transcription for each of the following words for which the lateral release in stop + /l/-clusters rule can apply.

cloud	kɫaʊd	**kˡlaʊd**	claʊd
plate	pʰleɪt	pɫeɪt	**pˡleɪt**
clue	kˡlue	**kˡlu**	kɫu
blow	**bˡloʊ**	blo	bɫoʊ
blade	**bˡleɪd**	bɫeɪd	bˡlade
glass	gɫæs	gˡlæss	**gˡlæs**
climb	kɫim	kˡlaɪmb	**kˡlaɪm**
glue	gˡɫu	gɫu	**gˡlu**
black	**bˡlæk**	bˡlæck	bɫæk
glove	gɫʌv	**gˡlʌv**	gɫʌve
clock	kˡlæk	kɫæk	**kˡlɑk**
pluck	pɫuk	pˡɫʌk	**pˡlʌk**

7–15. Stops: Transcribing Words With Affricated Alveolar Stops

Use narrow transcription to transcribe the following words, demonstrating allophonic affrication.

Word	Transcription
tree	t͡ʃɹi
dress	d͡ʒɹɛs
try	t͡ʃɹaɪ
dry	d͡ʒɹaɪ
tray	t͡ʃɹeɪ
drink	d͡ʒɹɪŋk
truck	t͡ʃɹʌk
drove	d͡ʒɹoʊv
metric	ˈmɛ.t͡ʃɹɪk
address	ˈæ.d͡ʒɹɛs - ə.ˈd͡ʒɹɛs

7–16. Stops: Transcribing Words With Word-Medial Taps

Pay attention to whether the medial stop is pronounced as /t/, /d/, or /ɾ/. Circle the words containing a tap phone. Then transcribe each word.

Word	Transcription
butter	ˈbʌ.ɾɚ
middle	ˈmɪ.ɾʊl
pretty	ˈpɹɪ.ɾi
valentine	ˈvæ.lən.taɪn
ladder	ˈlæ.ɾɚ
drumstick	ˈdɹʌm.stɪk

Word	Transcription
vitamin	ˈva͡ɪ.ɾə.mən
addendum	ə.ˈdɛn.dəm
military	ˈmɪ.lə.t͡ɛɚ.i
pity	ˈpɪ.ɾi
matter	ˈmæ.ɾɚ
hotel	ho͡ʊ.ˈtɛl
water	ˈwɑ.ɾɚ
addition	ə.ˈdɪ.ʃən
mighty	ˈma͡ɪ.ɾi
putter	ˈpʌ.ɾɚ
noodle	ˈnu.ɾəl
cactus	ˈkæk.təs
stutter	ˈstʌ.ɾɚ
litter	ˈlɪ.ɾɚ
sledding	ˈslɛ.ɾɪŋ
bathtub	ˈbæθ.təb
kitty	ˈkɪ.ɾi
address	ˈæ.dɹɛs
lunchtime	ˈlʌnt͡ʃ.ta͡ɪm
flighty	ˈfla͡ɪ.ɾi
photo	ˈfo͡ʊ.ɾo͡ʊ
spotty	ˈspɑ.ɾi

7–17. Stops: Identifying and Transcribing Utterances With Stop Shortening

Say each utterance aloud, paying attention to whether both stops in doubled contexts are fully articulated. Circle the word or phrase in each pair that contains a shortened stop in a doubled context. Then transcribe each word.

Utterance A	Utterance B	Transcription A	Transcription B
ribbing	**rib bone**	ˈɹɪ.bɪŋ	ɹɪb̚.bo͡ʊn
midday	middle	mɪd̚.de͡ɪ	ˈmɪ.ɾəl
lamppost	opposite	ˈlæmp̚.po͡ʊst	ˈɑ.pə.sɪt
sledding	**sled down**	ˈslɛ.ɾɪŋ	slɛd̚.da͡ʊn
cottage	**cattail**	ˈkɑ.ɹɪd͡ʒ	ˈkæt̚.te͡ɪl
subbasement	rabbit	sʌb̚.ˈbe͡ɪs.mənt	ˈɹæ.bɪt
adopt	**adduct**	ˈə.dɑpt	ˈæd̚.dəkt
crab bite	crabby	ˈkæb̚.ba͡ɪt	ˈkɹæ.bi
Let Tom.	lettuce	lɛt̚.tam	ˈlɛ.ɹəs
Stop it.	**Stop Pete.**	ˈstɑ.pɪt	stɑp̚.pit

7–18. Stops: Identifying Phrases With Glottal Stop Insertions

Circle the phrases that contain a glottal stop insertion between the vowels that end the first word and begin the second word.

roma apple	excellent ale	**angry alligator**
audio effect	icy icicle	**her heir**
busy alley	aqua sky	**shy ape**
edible egg	**my aide**	**bumpy avocado**
enter eagerly	**azalea aroma**	**heavy axle**

7–19. Stops: Identifying and Transcribing Words With Omission of /t/ in Word-Medial /nt/-Clusters

Circle the words for which the /t/ can be omitted in the word-medial /nt/-clusters. Then transcribe each word.

Word	Transcription
cantaloupe	ˈkæ.nə.lo͡ʊp
daughter	ˈdɔ.ɹɚ - ˈdɑ.ɹɚ
caterpillar	ˈkæ.ɹɚ.pɪ.lɚ
antibiotic	æ.na͡ɪ.ba͡ɪ.ˈɑ.ɹɪk
interesting	ɪ.nɚ.ˈɛ.stɪŋ
guitar	ɡɪ.ˈta͡ɚ
tomato	tə.ˈme͡ɪ.ɹo͡ʊ
twenty	ˈtwɛ.ni
beautiful	ˈbju.tə.fʊl - ˈbju.ɹə.fʊl
plentiful	ˈplɛ.nə.fʊl
computer	kəm.ˈpju.ɹɚ
hospital	ˈhɑ.spɪ.ɹʊl
winter	ˈwɪ.nɚ
vegetable	ˈvɛd͡ʒ.tə.bʊl
antonym	ˈæ.nə.nɪm
bountiful	ˈba͡ʊ.nə.fʊl
calculator	ˈka͡ʊl.kju.le͡ɪ.ɹɚ
internet	ˈɪ.nɚ.nɛt
entrance	ˈɛn.tɹəns

7–20. Fricatives: Transcribing Phrases With Palatalized /s/ and /z/

Use narrow transcription to transcribe the following words, all of which can be palatalized.

Phrase	Transcription
city's youth	sɪ.ɾi.ˈʒuθ
was young	wə.ˈʒəŋ
plus you	plə.ˈʃu
lose yourself	lu.ˈʒɝ.sɛlf
girls yearn	gɚl.ˈʒɝn
less yarn	lɛ.ˈʃa͡ɚn
this year	ðɪ.ˈʃi͡ɚ
egg's yolk	ɛg.ˈʒo͡ʊk
cars yield	ka͡ɚ.ˈʒild
use yeast	ju.ˈʒist
says yes	sɛ.ˈʒɛs
his yoyo	hɪ.ˈʒo͡ʊ.jo͡ʊ
the cab's yellow	ðə.kæb.ˈʒɛ.lo͡ʊ
Skip's yogurt	skɪp.ˈʒo͡ʊ.gɚt

7–21. Fricatives: Identifying Utterances With Devoicing of [v] in /v/ + Voiceless Consonant Contexts

Circle the phrases for which the devoicing of [v] in /v/ + voiceless consonant contexts rule can apply.

have fun	behave yourself	**wave hello**
arrive late	**love phonetics**	**five trees**
give thanks	**move quickly**	**save face**
dive shallow	**pave streets**	**drive far**
above board	**shave carefully**	believe now
remove doubt	**thrive today**	**festive party**
improve now	twelve boys	**live free**

7–22. Fricatives: Identifying and Transcribing Words With Voiced [s] in Voiced Consonant + /s/ Contexts

Say each word aloud, paying attention to voicing of [s] in voiced consonant + /s/ contexts. Circle the words containing voiced [s] (that is, [z]). Then transcribe each word.

Word A	Word B	Transcription A	Transcription B
pats	**pans**	pæts	pænz
dogs	dots	dɔgz - dɑgz	dɑts
harms	hearths	hɑɚmz	hɑɚθs
jobs	jocks	d͡ʒɑbz	d͡ʒɑks
wicks	**whims**	wɪks	wɪmz
falls	faults	fɔlz - fɑlz	fɑlts
buys	bites	ba͡ɪz	ba͡ɪts
heats	**heeds**	hits	hidz
woks	**watches**	wɑks	ˈwɑ.t͡ʃəz
foals	folks	fo͡ʊlz	fo͡ʊlks

7–23. Fricatives: Identifying and Transcribing Words With Fricative Lengthening

Say each utterance aloud, paying attention to whether both fricatives in doubled contexts are lengthened. Circle the utterances containing fricative lengthening. Then transcribe each word.

Utterance A	Utterance B	Transcription A	Transcription B
caffeine	**calf feed**	kæ.ˈfin	kæfːid
his zipper	unzip	hɪzːɪ.pɚ	ən.ˈzɪp
guesser	**yes sir**	ˈgɛ.sɚ	jɛsːɚ
buff feet	buffy	bʌfːit	ˈbʌ.fi
buses	**bus seat**	ˈbʌsːəz	bʌsːit
cat's skills	Catskills	kætsːkɪlz	kæt.skɪlz
stuff fell	stuffing	stəfːɛl	ˈstʌ.fɪŋ
alphabet	**half phase**	ˈæl.fə.bɛt	hæfːeɪz
password	**misspell**	ˈpæs.wɚd	mɪˈsːpɛl
graffiti	**graph fuel**	gɹə.ˈfi.ɾi	gɹæfːjul

7–24. Fricatives: Identifying Phrases With Omission of /h/ in Unstressed Contexts

Circle the phrases that can contain omission of /h/ in unstressed contexts.

Let's have FUN!   **Look him in the EYES.**

HE's a jolly good fellow.   **WHICH way did he go?**

PLEASE, give me her number.   Do YOU know who's going?

YOU have to HELP me.   We HAD to run fast.

I like HER attitude.   **See how much it COSTS.**

7–25. Affricates: Identifying and Transcribing Words With Labialized Affricates

Say each word aloud, paying attention to whether the affricate preceding the vowel is labialized rule can apply. Circle the words containing a labialized affricate. Then transcribe each word.

Word	Transcription
choke	t͡ʃʷo͡ʊk
cheek	t͡ʃik
chew	t͡ʃʷu
jive	d͡ʒa͡ɪv
juice	d͡ʒʷus
jaw	d͡ʒʷɔ - d͡ʒɑ
matches	ˈmæ.t͡ʃəz
nachos	ˈnɑ.t͡ʃʷo͡ʊz
ketchup	ˈkɛ.t͡ʃəp
pitcher	ˈpɪ.t͡ʃʷɚ
major	ˈme͡ɪ.d͡ʒʷɚ
apologize	ə.ˈpɑ.lə.d͡ʒa͡ɪz
soldier	ˈso͡ʊl.d͡ʒʷɚ

7–26. Nasals: Identifying and Transcribing Utterances With Labiodentalized /m/

1. Circle the utterances for which the labiodentalized /m/ rule can apply.

ham for dinner	**some flowers**	amphitheater
phone family	**emphasize**	**swam fast**
ephemeral	**swim fast**	**palm fronds**
harrumph	same friends	**triumphant**
film violence	**from Venus**	broken vase

2. All the following words can contain a labiodentalized /m/. Transcribe each word.

symphonic	sɪm̪.ˈfɑ.nɪk
camphor	ˈkæm̪.fɚ
amphibian	æm̪.ˈfɪ.bi.ən
emphatic	ɛm̪.ˈfæ.ɾɪk
Humvee	həm̪.ˈvi
circumvent	sɚ.kəm̪.ˈvɛnt

7–27. Nasals: Identifying and Transcribing Words With Velarized /n/

Read the following sets of words aloud, paying attention to whether the *n* sounds are produced as /n/, /ŋ/, or /ŋk/. Then transcribe each word.

thin	θɪn	think	θɪŋk	thing	θɪŋ
sin	sɪn	sink	sɪŋk	sing	sɪŋ
win	wɪn	wink	wɪŋk	wing	wɪŋ
ran	ɹæn	rank	ɹæŋk	rang	ɹæŋ
clan	klæn	clank	klæŋk	clang	klæŋ
stun	stʌn	stunk	stʌŋk	stung	stʌŋ
tan	tæn	tank	tæŋk	tang	tæŋ
angel	ˈeɪn.d͡ʒəl	ankle	ˈæŋ.kəl	angle	ˈæŋ.gəl
tongue	tʌŋ	singing	ˈsɪŋ.ɪŋ		
blanket	ˈblæŋ.kət	thinking	ˈθɪŋ.kɪŋ		
trinket	ˈtɹɪŋ.kət	unkind	ˈən.ka͡ɪnd		
hanger	ˈhæŋ.ɚ	angelic	æn.ˈd͡ʒɛ.lɪk		

7–28. Nasals: Identifying and Transcribing Utterances With Nasal Lengthening

Say each utterance aloud, paying attention to whether both nasals in doubled contexts are lengthened. Circle the utterances containing nasal lengthening. Then transcribe each utterance.

Utterance A	Utterance B	Transcription A	Transcription B
hammered	**from Mars**	ˈhæ.mɚd	fɹəmːɑɚ̯z
swim meet	swimmer	ˈswɪmːit	ˈswɪ.mɚ
running	**Run now.**	ˈɹʌ.nɪŋ	ɹʌnːaʊ̯
unplanned	**openness**	ən.ˈplænd	ˈoʊ̯.pənːəs
unnerve	announce	ənːˈɝv	ə.ˈnaʊ̯nts
brownnoser	annex	ˈbɹaʊ̯nːoʊ̯.zɚ	ˈæ.nɛks
summer	**some money**	ˈsʌ.mɚ	sʌmːˈʌ.ni
unnatural	penny	ʌnːˈæ.t͡ʃɚ.əl	ˈpɛ.ni
tenderness	**thinness**	ˈtɛn.dɚ.nəs	ˈθɪnː.əs
nonnative	annihilate	nɑnːˈeɪ̯.ɾɪv	ə.ˈnaɪ̯.ɪ.le͡ɪt

7–29. Nasals: Identifying and Transcribing Words With Syllabic Nasals

Pay attention to whether the word-final nasal is syllabic. Circle the words containing syllabic nasals. Then transcribe each word.

Word	Transcription
awaken	ə.ˈweɪ.k̚n̩
Amazon	ˈæ.mə.zɑn
summon	ˈsʌ.mn̩
magazine	ˈmæ.gə.zin
explain	ɛk.ˈspleɪn
urban	ˈɝ.bn̩
imprison	m̩.ˈpɹɪ.zn̩
listen	ˈlɪ.sn̩
ma'am	ˈmæm
burden	ˈbɝ.d̄n̩
prism	ˈpɹɪ.zm̩
column	ˈkɑ.lm̩

7–30. Nasals: Identifying and Transcribing Words With Nasal Lengthening and Syllabification

Say each word aloud to determine if there is evidence of nasal lengthening and/or nasal syllabification. Phonetically transcribe each word. Mark an X in the appropriate box. Then describe the reason for this type of assimilation. The first one has been done for you.

Word	Phonetic Transcription	Syllabic	Lengthened	Description
mission	ˈmɪ.ʃn̩	X		The weak vowel can be eliminated and replaced by a syllabic consonant, which acts as the nucleus of the syllable.
evenness	ˈi.vənːɛs		X	A consonant is articulated for a longer duration than that of a corresponding nondoubled consonant.
rhythm	ˈɹɪ.ðm̩	X		The weak vowel can be eliminated and replaced by a syllabic consonant, which acts as the nucleus of the syllable.
important	m̩.ˈpɔɚ.tʰənt	X		The weak vowel can be eliminated and replaced by a syllabic consonant, which acts as the nucleus of the syllable.
roommate	ˈɹum̩ːeɪtʰ		X	A consonant is articulated for a longer duration than that of a corresponding nondoubled consonant.
indeed	n̩.ˈdid	X		The weak vowel can be eliminated and replaced by a syllabic consonant, which acts as the nucleus of the syllable.
team mascot	timːæ.skɑt		X	A consonant is articulated for a longer duration than that of a corresponding nondoubled consonant.

7–31. Approximants: Transcribing Words With Dark-l in Post-Vocalic Contexts

Each of the following words contains a dark-l in post-vocalic position. Transcribe each word.

Word	Transcription
fault	fɔɫt / fɑɫt
coal	ko͡ʊɫ
film	fɪɫm
wilt	wɪɫt
mail	me͡ɪɫ
bells	bɛɫz
guilt	gɪɫt
balk	bɑɫk
elm	ɛɫm
soil	sɔ͡ɪɫ

7–32. Approximants: Identifying and Transcribing Words With Devoiced /w, j, l, ɹ/ in Voiceless Stop + Approximant Clusters

Circle the words containing a devoiced approximant as a result of the voiceless stop + approximant clusters rule. Then transcribe each word.

Word A	Word B	Transcription A	Transcription B
pew	beauty	pju̥	bju.ɾi
pajamas	**pupil**	ˈpə.d͡ʒæ.məz	ˈpju̥.pəl
apply	apple	ə.ˈpl̥a͡ɪ	ˈæ.pəl
plaid	bladder	pl̥æd	ˈblæ.dɚ
beetle	**between**	ˈbi.ɾəl	bi.ˈtw̥in
dry	**try**	dɹa͡ɪ	tɹ̥a͡ɪ
matron	matter	ˈme͡ɪ.tɹ̥ən	ˈmæ.ɾɚ
acquire	squire	ə.ˈkw̥a͡ɪɚ	skwa͡ɪɚ
aghast	**acute**	ə.ˈgæst	ə.ˈkj̥ut
cyclops	blot	ˈsa͡ɪ.kl̥aps	blɑt
acrid	grand	ˈæ.kɹ̥ɪd	ˈgɹænd

7–33. Approximants: Identifying Phrases With Lengthened /l/

Circle the phrases that typically contain lengthening of /l/ in double /l/ contexts.

pearl locket	pal around	**goal line**
pencil lines	mole hill	tell her
full laundry	**girl laughing**	**football locker**
bill due	pal around	**tall ladder**
grill out	pole vaulter	**small lock**
sell land	heavy lifting	live life

7–34. Approximants: Identifying and Transcribing Words With Syllabic /l/ in Unstressed Word-Final Contexts

Circle the words for which the final /l/ can be syllabified in unstressed word-final contexts. Then transcribe each word.

Word	Transcription
final	ˈfaɪ.nl̩
nickel	ˈnɪ.kl̩
bottle	ˈbɑ.ɾl̩
jackal	ˈd͡ʒæ.kl̩
needle	ˈni.dl̩
hill	ˈhɪl
finial	ˈfɪ.ni.l̩
peel	ˈpil
silt	ˈsɪlt
saddle	ˈsæ.ɾl̩
shelf	ˈʃɛlf

7–35. Narrow Transcription of Sentences

Apply as many diacritics as you can to narrowly transcribe the following sentences!

	Sentence	Transcription
1.	The cats scattered.	ðə kʰæts sk⁼æ.ɹɚd
2.	Please tell the truth.	pˡl̥iz̥ tɛɬ ðə t͡ʃɹuθ
3.	Do you want the cute puppy?	dʷu ju wan̪t̪ ðə kʷjuˀ 'pʰʌ.pi
4.	The garden died last winter.	ðə 'gɑɚ̯dⁿ.n̩ dɑɪd læst̚ 'wɪ.nɚ
5.	Escape cold weather today.	ə.'sk⁼e͡ɪpˀ ko͡ʊɫd 'wɛ.ðɚ tʰu.'de͡ɪ

8

VOWEL PHONOLOGY

8–1. Identifying and Transcribing Stressed and Unstressed Schwa and Wedge

Each of the following highlighted words has at least one vowel produced with a schwa and/ or a wedge. Underline the syllable (or syllables) that contain a wedge or a schwa. Put a check in the appropriate column if the word contains a schwa, wedge, or a schwa and a wedge. Then transcribe the word, marking the stressed vowel with an apostrophe at the beginning of the syllable.

	Word	/ʌ/	/ə/	Phonetic Transcription
1.	salami		x	sə.ˈlɑ.mi
2.	buffalo	x	x	ˈbʌ.fə.loʊ
3.	enough	x	x	ə.ˈnʌf
4.	detect		x	də.ˈtɛkt
5.	between		x	bə.ˈtwin
6.	united		x	ju.ˈnaɪ.ɾəd
7.	televise		x	ˈtɛ.lə.vaɪz
8.	sunny	x		ˈsʌ.ni
9.	pumice	x		ˈpʌ.mɪs
10.	customary	x	x	ˈkʌs.tə.mɛ˞.i

8–2. Identifying Schwa /ə/ and Wedge /ʌ/

For each of the following highlighted words, use the table to mark with an "X" which of the target words contains a schwa /ə/, wedge /ʌ/, both, or neither. Then transcribe the word.

Target Word	Wedge	Schwa	Both	Neither	Transcription
muffin	X				ˈmʌ.fɪn
can				X	kæn
bucket	X				ˈbʌ.kɪt
malice				X	ˈmæ.lɪs
luck	X				lʌk
unique				X	ju.ˈnik
above			X		ə.ˈbʌv
beauty				X	ˈbju.ɾi
forest		X			ˈfɔɚ.əst
stomach	X				ˈstʌ.mɪk
syringe		X			sə.ˈɹɪndʒ
none	X				nʌn
mend				X	mɛnd
love	X				lʌv
summit	X				ˈsʌ.mɪt
cup	X				kʌp
data		X			ˈdæ.ɾə
divide				X	dɪ.ˈvaɪd
oven			X		ˈʌ.vən
cut	X				kʌt

Target Word	Wedge	Schwa	Both	Neither	Transcription
emphasize		X			ˈɛm.fə.saɪz
puppet			X		ˈpʌ.pət
sash				X	sæʃ
muddy	X				ˈmʌ.ɾi
cupboard	X				ˈkʌ.bɚd
sofa		X			ˈsoʊ.fə
troops				X	tɹups
adore		X			ə.ˈdɔɚ

8–3. Identifying Stressed and Unstressed Vowels: /ʌ/ and /ə/

Each of the following words contain the wedge /ʌ/ or the schwa /ə/. Circle the words that are most frequently produced with the unstressed schwa /ə/.

bunny	tub	**jacket**
bug	**ocean**	cut
sofa	fun	**passion**
dumb	shun	**ability**
come	**about**	cup
love	**ago**	**token**
silent	bus	**system**
plunge	**reason**	**harmony**
parrot	**bottom**	luck
welcome	done	rut

8–4. Transcribing Mid Central Vowel Stressed and Unstressed Allophonic Variations

Transcribe each highlighted multisyllabic word, capturing production differences of the mid central vowel with [ʌ] or [ə].

1. umbrella   [əm.ˈbɹɛ.lə]

2. mud   [mʌd]

3. tongue   [tʌŋ]

4. complete   [kəm.ˈplit]

5. donut   [ˈdo͡ʊ.nət]

6. what   [wʌt]

7. rough   [ɹʌf]

8. deduced   [də.ˈdust]

9. welcome   [ˈwɛɫ.kəm]

10. lunch   [lʌnt͡ʃ]

11. rusty   [ˈɹʌ.sti]

12. alone   [ə.ˈlo͡ʊn]

13. done   [dʌn]

14. provide   [ˈpɹə.va͡ɪd]

15. plumbing   [ˈplʌ.mɪŋ]

16. describe   [də.ˈskɹa͡ɪb]

8–5. Identifying and Transcribing Stressed and Unstressed Schwar

Each word has at least one vowel produced with stressed or unstressed schwar. Say the high-lighted multisyllabic words aloud. Circle the syllable (or syllables) that contains a stressed or unstressed schwar. Put a check in the appropriate column if the word contains a stressed shwar, an unstressed schwar, or a stressed and an unstressed schwar. Then transcribe the word.

	Word	/ɝ/	/ɚ/	Phonetic Transcription
1.	<u>sur</u>prise		x	sɚ.ˈpɹaɪz
2.	runn<u>er</u>		x	ˈɹʌ.nɚ
3.	<u>bur</u>ning	x		ˈbɝ.nɪŋ
4.	stutt<u>ered</u>		x	ˈstʌ.ɾɚd
5.	thund<u>er</u>		x	ˈθʌn.dɚ
6.	<u>cour</u>teous	x		ˈkɝ.ɾi.əs
7.	<u>pur</u>ple	x		ˈpɝ.pəl
8.	<u>fur</u>ry	x		ˈfɝ.i
9.	<u>for</u>giveness		x	fɚ.ˈgɪv.nɪs
10.	custom<u>er</u>		x	ˈkʌs.tə.mɚ

8–6. Vowel Nasalization

Circle the following words that contain a nasalized vowel.

window **thing** arithmetic

alarm **bean** hammer

potato **crown** mouth

ring adult pillow

tongue nose **computer**

bookcase **storm** river

drum kidney **moon**

8–7. Vowel Tenseness

Circle the words that contain a lax vowel.

cat	**sit**	boot
bell	**hook**	pond
nut	comb	**tin**
bet	sock	mouse
watch	**sand**	nail
beard	**dress**	**push**

8–8. Capturing Vowel Length

In each of the following word pairs, circle the word with the longer vowel according to rules for vowel length in English. Transcribe both words using narrow transcription and diacritics to capture the vowel length difference.

Word Pair		Narrow Transcription	
safe	**save**	seͪf	seͪːv
lock	**log**	lɑˑk	lɑːg
see	seating	siː	ˈsiˑ.ɾɪŋ
two	tool	tuː	tuˑɫ
beat	**bead**	biˑt	biːd
set	settle	sɛːt	ˈsɛˑ.təɫ
team	**tea**	tiˑm	tiː
cab	cap	kæːb	kæˑp

8–9. Vowel Length

Circle the word in each word pair that, according to typical phonological patterns of English, will contain a longer vowel.

suit	**sued**
play	plate
pea	peak
bit	bitter
trapper	**trap**
bet	**bed**
row	wrote
plot	**dog**
joy	void
shook	**should**

8–10. Vowel Length in Stressed Versus Unstressed Syllables

The following words are presented in pairs. Transcribe both words. A syllable in each word contains the same phonemes. Circle the word where the matching syllable would be longer. If the syllables will be the same length, circle both words. Remember that for /ʌ/ and /ɝ/, stress distinctions can be captured with allophonic symbols [ə] and [ɚ].

1.	fasten	**sunny**	ˈfæ.sən	ˈsʌ.ni
2.	**into**	intact	ˈɪn.tu	ɪn.ˈtækt
3.	**catsup**	bobcat	ˈkæt.səp	bɑb.kæt
4.	**current**	**recur**	ˈkɝ.ənt	ɹə.ˈkɝ
5.	**delete**	athlete	də.ˈlit	ˈæθ.lit
6.	coughing	**finger**	ˈkɑ.fɪŋ	ˈfɪŋ.gɚ
7.	urbane	**purring**	ˈɚ.ˈbeɪn	ˈpɝ.ɪŋ
8.	**admit**	summit	əd.ˈmɪt	ˈsʌ.mɪt
9.	**gulping**	beagle	ˈgʌl.pɪŋ	ˈbi.gəɫ
10.	**support**	**portly**	sə.ˈpɔɚt	ˈpɔɚt.li

8–11. Vowel Length

Put the following words in order based on length of vowel production in each of them (longest to shortest). Assume the only difference in vowel length is based on English phonological patterns.

/i/   knead   sheet   bee   mosquito
bee, knead, sheet, mosquito

/ɪ/   ability   bigger   kiss   dig
dig, kiss, bigger, ability

/ʊ/   neighborhood   put   should   rookie
should, put, rookie, neighborhood

/aɪ/   type   excite   bye   excitement
bye, type, excite, excitement

/u/   January   computer   views   compute
views, compute, computer, January

/e/   state   bathe   locate   location
bathe, state, locate, location

/ɛ/   net   education   red   better
red, net, better, education

/aʊ/   cloud   cow   flower   shout
cow, cloud, shout, flower

/oʊ/   roam   show   devote   soap
show, roam, soap, devote

/ʌ/   independence   alert   tub   summer
tub, summer, alert, independence

8–12. Coarticulation

For each word in the following chart, describe in detail the type of anticipatory and/or carryover coarticulation that will likely occur on the vowel. Then transcribe the word, using narrow transcription to capture the coarticulation.

Word	Description	Narrow Transcription
1. spoon	[u] is nasalized because it occurs before a nasal consonant.	spũn
2. basketball	[a] is retracted because it is produced before a velar [ɫ].	ˈbæ.skɪt.bɑɫ
3. install	[ɪ] is nasalized because it follows a nasal consonant. [a] is retracted because it is produced before a velar [ɫ].	ĭn.ˈstɑɫ
4. architect	[ɪ] is devoiced because it occurs after a voiceless consonant in an unstressed syllable.	ˈɑɚ.kɪ̥.tɛkt
5. tropical	[ə] is retracted because it is before a velar [ɫu]. [a] is partially rounded because it is preceded by an [ɹ].	ˈtɹɑ.pɪ.kə̣ɫ
6. rebel	[ə] is retracted because it is before a velar [ɫ].	ˈɹɛ.bə̣ɫ
7. sprain	The [eɪ] is nasalized because it is before a nasal consonant.	spɹẽɪ̃n
8. wrong	[a] is nasalized because it is before a nasal consonant.	ɹɑ̃ŋ
9. win	[ɪ] is nasalized because it is before a nasal consonant.	wɪ̃n
10. still	[ɪ] is retracted because it is before a velar [ɫ].	stɪ̠ɫ

8–13. Transcription Errors

Which of the following transcriptions contain an error? Mark C for correct and I for incorrect. If incorrect, transcribe the word correctly.

chapter	t͡ʃæpdɛɚ	I	ˈt͡ʃæp.dɚ
grain	gɹaɪn	I	gɹeɪn
push	puʃ	C	
plate	pleɪt	C	
desk	dɛsk	C	
boat	boʊt	C	
phone	fɔn	I	foʊn
dot	dat	I	dat
rain	ɹæn	I	ɹeɪn
pie	pi	I	paɪ
boy	bɔɪ	C	
cloud	kloʊd	I	klaʊd
bird	bɝd	C	
leaf	lɛf	I	lif
mop	mɑp	C	
feel	fil	C	
sun	sən	I	sʌn
kit	kɪt	C	
bus	bʌs	C	
rat	ɹɑt	I	ɹæt

8–14. Diacritic Use

Each of the following words contain a diacritic providing additional information about the vowel. Circle "correct" if the diacritic correctly describes General American English vowel phonological patterns. Circle "incorrect" if the diacritic is not used correctly.

stɹi̥t	**Correct**	Incorrect
dɹĩŋk	**Correct**	Incorrect
tɹiː	**Correct**	Incorrect
ˈbɑ̩.ɹəl	Correct	**Incorrect**
ˈwʊ.mə̃n	**Correct**	Incorrect
ˈpɛn.sə̣ɫ	Correct	**Incorrect**
hɪ̥ɫ	**Correct**	Incorrect
ˈpæ.kə̃t	Correct	**Incorrect**
bɹɪ̥k	**Correct**	Incorrect

8–15. Identifying Accurate Narrow Transcription

Circle the best narrow transcription of the following words.

1.	topography	tʰə.ˈpʰɑ̣.ɡɹə.fi	(tʰə.ˈpʰɑ.ɡɹə.fi)	tʰə.ˈpʰɑ.ɡɹə.fi̥
2.	sheet	(ʃi̥t˺)	ʃĩt˺	ʃi̥t˺
3.	name	nei̥m	nei̥m	(neĩm)
4.	telephone	ˈtʰɛ.lə.foʊ̃n	(ˈtʰɛ.lə.foʊ̃n)	ˈtɛ.lə.foʊ̥n
5.	feel	(fiɫ)	fĩl	fĩl
6.	potato	pʰə.ˈtʰeɪ.ɾoʊ	pʰə.ˈtʰeɪ.ɾoʊ̥	(pʰə̣.ˈtʰeɪ.ɾoʊ)
7.	monkey	(ˈmʌ̃ŋ.kʰĩ)	ˈmʌŋ.kʰĩ	ˈmʌŋ.kʰi
8.	shadow	ˈʃæʰ.ɾoʊ	(ˈʃæ.ɾoʊ)	ˈʃæ.ɾoʊ
9.	catastrophe	kʰə.ˈtʰæ.stɹə.fi	kʰə.ˈtʰæ.stɹə.fi̥	(kʰə.ˈtʰæ.stɹə.fi)
10.	ring	(ɹĩŋ)	ɹi̥ŋ	ɹi̥ŋ
11.	track	(tɹ̥æk)	tɹ̥æ̈k	tɹ̥æk
12.	drip	dɹɪ̃ʷp	dɹɪ̈p	(dɹɪ̥p)

8–16. Narrow Transcription

Say aloud. Transcribe the highlighted words, using diacritics to differentiate vowel length and vowel stress patterns.

listen	[ˈlɪː.sɪn]
currently	[ˈkɝː.ĕnˌliˑ]
attitude	[ˈaː.ɾĭˌtʊˑd]
council	[ˈka͡ʊːn.səɫ]
obvious	[ˈaːb.ˌviˑ.ə̆s]
union	[ˈjuːn.jən]
again	[əˈgɛːn]
impossible	[ĭmˈpaː.sĭˌbəˑɫ]
downhill	[ˈda͡ʊːn.hɪɫ]
musical	[ˈmjuː.zĭˌkəˑɫ]
persuasive	[pɚˈswe͡ɪːˌsɪˑv]
another	[ə̆ˈnʌː.ðɚˑ]
education	[ˌɛˑ.ʤə̆ˈke͡ɪː.ʃə̆n]
destroying	[də̆ˈstɔ͡ɪːˌɹˑɪŋ]
mathematics	[ˌmæˑ.θə̆ˈmæː.ɾə̆ks]
communication	[kə̆ˌmjuˑ.nĭˈke͡ɪː.ʃə̆n]

BEYOND GENERAL AMERICAN ENGLISH
Speech Possibilities Within and Across Languages

9–1. Language Terms

Complete the following definitions with the correct term.

1. A person who uses more than two languages is called a **multilingual**.

2. Mutually intelligible variants of a language are called **dialects**.

3. The predecessor of all languages in a language family is a **protolanguage**.

4. Related languages that share linguistic properties belong to a **language family**.

5. A person who uses two languages is called **a bilingual**.

6. A language used by people to communicate when they do not share the same first language is called a **lingua franca**.

7. A community's shared communication of words and rules for combining and producing words is called a **language**.

8. Dialects that trace back to a geographic region are called **regional dialects**.

9. Dialects that are shared by individuals identifying as a subgroup of a community are called **social dialects**.

9–2. Identifying Active and Passive Articulators

Determine if the following places of articulation are active or passive and upper or lower surface.

1.	Tongue front	**active lower surface**
2.	Hard palate	**passive upper surface**
3.	Alveolar ridge	**passive upper surface**
4.	Tongue root	**active lower surface**
5.	Lower lip	**active lower surface**
6.	Pharyngeal wall	**passive upper surface**
7.	Post-alveolar region	**passive upper surface**
8.	Soft palate	**passive upper surface**
9.	Tongue back	**active lower surface**
10.	Tongue blade	**active lower surface**
11.	Underside of the tongue	**active lower surface**
12.	Upper lip	**active upper surface**
13.	Uvula	**passive upper surface**
14.	Tongue tip	**active lower surface**

9–3. Identifying Pulmonic Consonants

Circle yes or no to indicate whether the place, manner, and voicing combinations are phonemic in English. Transcribe the phoneme.

		Phonemic in English?	Phonetic Transcription
1.	voiced uvular stop	Yes / **No**	/ɢ/
2.	voiced labiodental nasal	Yes / **No**	/ɱ/
3.	voiced dental fricative	**Yes** / No	/ð/
4.	voiceless glottal stop	Yes / **No**	/ʔ/ (allophonic, not phonemic, in English)
5.	voiced bilabial trill	Yes / **No**	/ʙ/
6.	voiced retroflex flap	Yes / **No**	/ɽ/
7.	voiceless palatal stop	Yes / **No**	/c/
8.	voiced lateral palatal liquid	Yes / **No**	/ʎ/
9.	voiceless velar fricative	Yes / **No**	/x/
10.	voiced palatal fricative	Yes / **No**	/ʝ/
11.	voiced palatal approximant glide	**Yes** / No	/j/
12.	voiced uvular nasal	Yes / **No**	/ɴ/

9–4. Airstream Terminology

Complete the following definitions with the correct term.

1. If a speech sound is produced when air is leaving the vocal tract, it is produced on an **egressive** airstream.

2. If a speech sound is produced when air is rushing into the vocal tract, it is produced on an **ingressive** airstream.

3. The airstream source for a click is **velaric.**

4. The airstream source for an ejective is **glottalic.**

5. The airstream source for a plosive is **pulmonic.**

6. A speech sound made on a velaric ingressive airstream is called a(n) **click.**

7. A speech sound made on a glottalic egressive airstream is called a(n) **ejective.**

8. A speech sound made on a pulmonic egressive airstream is called a(n) **plosive.**

9. A speech sound made on a glottalic ingressive airstream is called a(n) **implosive.**

9–5. Airstreams Used in Speech Production

Which airstream source and direction is used to make each of the following sounds?

1. Click   **velaric ingressive**

2. Ejective   **glottalic egressive**

3. Nasal   **pulmonic egressive**

4. Plosive   **pulmonic egressive**

5. Fricative   **pulmonic egressive**

6. Implosive   **glottalic ingressive**

7. Vowel   **pulmonic egressive**

8. Liquid   **pulmonic egressive**

9–6. Non-Pulmonic Sounds

Write the articulatory characterizations for the following non-pulmonic IPA symbols (voicing, place, and manner). An example has been done for you.

1. /ǃk/   voiceless postalveolar click

2. /ǂŋ/   nasal palatal click

3. /p'/   voiceless bilabial ejective

4. /ǀk/   voiceless dental click

5. /ʘg/   voiced bilabial click

6. /ʙ/   voiced bilabial trill

7. /ʜ/   voiceless epiglottal fricative

8. /ɗ/   voiced alveolar implosive

9. /t'/   voiceless alveolar ejective

10. /β/   voiced bilabial fricative

11. /ɠ/   voiced velar implosive

12. /ɮ/   voiced lateral fricative

13. /ɬ/   voiceless lateral fricative

14. /ǁg/   voiced lateral click

9–7. Airflow

Identify whether each phoneme has an egressive or ingressive airflow. Circle the correct answer.

1. /k'/   a) ingressive   b) **egressive**

2. /ɓ/   a) **ingressive**   b) egressive

3. /m/   a) ingressive   b) **egressive**

4. /ʘg/   a) **ingressive**   b) egressive

5. /ɢ/   a) **ingressive**   b) egressive

6. /s'/   a) ingressive   b) **egressive**

7. /w/   a) ingressive   b) **egressive**

8. /ǂŋ/   a) **ingressive**   b) egressive

9. /ɗ/   a) **ingressive**   b) egressive

10. /ǃk/   a) **ingressive**   b) egressive

9–8. Describing and Contrasting Sounds Across Languages

The following times indicate different voice onset time (VOT) delays. Match these possible VOT delays with the type of plosive consonant.

                    –20 ms   0 ms   40 ms   80 ms

Strongly aspirated stop   **80 ms**

Voiceless unaspirated stop   **0 ms**

Fully voiced stop   **–20 ms**

Slightly aspirated stop   **40 ms**

9–9. Describing Consonants

You were introduced to nine ways that consonants can differ. These are (1) airstream source, (2) airstream direction, (3) state of glottis, (4) part of tongue (can be NA), (5) place, (6) centrality, (7) nasality, (8) manner, and (9) length. Define the nine categories for each of the following sounds.

1. /p'/
1) glottalic
2) egressive
3) voiceless
4) NA
5) bilabial
6) central
7) oral
8) ejective
9) singleton

2. /‖ŋ/
1) velaric
2) ingressive
3) voiced
4) apical
5) alveolar
6) lateral
7) nasal
8) click
9) singleton

3. /ʄː/
1) glottalic
2) ingressive
3) voiced
4) laminal
5) palatal
6) central
7) oral
8) implosive
9) geminate

4. /ɢ/
1) pulmonic
2) egressive
3) creaky
4) dorsal
5) uvular
6) central
7) oral
8) plosive
9) singleton

5. /d̪/
1) pulmonic
2) egressive
3) breathy
4) apical
5) alveolar
6) central
7) oral
8) plosive
9) singleton

6. /ʙː/
1) pulmonic
2) egressive
3) voiced
4) NA
5) bilabial
6) central
7) oral
8) trill
9) geminate

7. /ɭ/
1) pulmonic
2) egressive
3) voiced
4) apical
5) retroflex
6) lateral
7) oral
8) approximant
9) singleton

8. /t͡s'/   1) glottalic   2) egressive   3) voiceless
            4) apical   5) alveolar   6) central
            7) oral   8) affricate ejective 9) singleton

9–10. Speech Sound Inventories

The following are contrived vowel and consonant inventories for different languages. Note whether these inventories are likely or unlikely and why.

1. Language A Vowels: /i, ɪ, y, ʏ, ɛ, e, æ/

   Unlikely. All vowels are front vowels and there is not enough perceptual distance between them.

2. Language B Vowels: /i, e, ɑ, o, u/

   Likely. These five vowels are perceptually distinct and involve simple articulatory movements. This is a common five-vowel inventory.

3. Language C Vowels: /i, e̞, a͡ɪ, õ, uː/

   Unlikely. These vowels do not need to be so complex to produce to have adequate perceptual distance in a five-vowel language system.

4. Language D Vowels: /i, e, ɛ/

   Unlikely. While basic vowels and easy to produce, their acoustic qualities are very similar thus they do not maximize perceptual distinctiveness.

5. Language A Consonants: /ɴ, ʕ, ʀ, ʈ͡ʂ, ʟ/

   Unlikely. These sounds are elaborated consonants. Languages typically maximize basic consonants before adding elaborated consonants for greater perceptual contrast.

6. Language B Consonants: /d, g, b, m, n, s, f, j/

   Likely. These are basic consonants. There are stops, nasals, glides, and fricatives. They provide substantial perceptual contrast for a smaller consonant inventory.

10

TRANSCRIPTION PRACTICE

10–1. Single-Syllable Words: 1

1. *back*   [bæk]

2. *time*   [t͡aɪm]

3. *jump*   [d͡ʒʌmp]

4. *rogue*   [ɹo͡ʊg]

5. *shield*   [ʃiɫd]

6. *tone*   [to͡ʊn]

7. *breathe*   [bɹið]

8. *church*   [t͡ʃɝt͡ʃ]

9. *guest*   [gɛst]

10. *bathe*   [be͡ɪð]

11. *hook*   [hʊk]

12. *globe*   [glo͡ʊb]

10–2. Single-Syllable Words: 2

1. *think*   [θɪŋk]

2. *scream*   [skɹim]

3. *down*   [da͡ʊn]

4. *oak*   [o͡ʊk]

5. *beef*   [bif]

6. *shake*   [ʃe͡ɪk]

7. *missed*   [mɪst]

8. *beige*   [be͡ɪʒ]

9. *sheep*   [ʃip]

10. *lunch*   [lʌnt͡ʃ]

11. *smooth*   [smuð]

12. *count*   [ka͡ʊnt]

10–3. Single-Syllable Words: 3

1. *date*   [de͡ɪt]

2. *curb*   [kɝb]

3. *eat*   [it]

4. *cheese*   [t͡ʃiz]

5. *few*   [fju]

6. *this*   [ðɪs]

7. *was*   [wʌz]

8. *yolk*   [jo͡ʊk]

9. *vowel*   [va͡ʊɫ]

10. *zest*   [zɛst]

11. *blaze*   [ble͡ɪz]

12. *shine*   [ʃa͡ɪn]

10–4. Single-Syllable Words: 4

1. *thank* [θæŋk]

2. *dwell* [dwɛɫ]

3. *reach* [ɹit͡ʃ]

4. *yard* [jɑɚd]

5. *trust* [tɹʌst]

6. *mesh* [mɛʃ]

7. *dish* [dɪʃ]

8. *fly* [flaɪ]

9. *shut* [ʃʌt]

10. *boot* [but]

11. *moon* [mun]

12. *theft* [θɛft]

10–5. Single-Syllable Words: 5

1. *month*   [mʌnθ]

2. *sign*   [sa͡ɪn]

3. *latch*   [læt͡ʃ]

4. *shrink*   [ʃɹɪŋk]

5. *zoo*   [zu]

6. *booth*   [buθ]

7. *those*   [ðo͡ʊz]

8. *theft*   [θɛft]

9. *shrimp*   [ʃɹɪmp]

10. *ledge*   [lɛd͡ʒ]

11. *stretch*   [stɹɛt͡ʃ]

12. *wait*   [we͡ɪt]

10–6. Single-Syllable Words: 6

1. *boss*   [bɑs]

2. *spring*   [spɹɪŋ]

3. *vague*   [veɪɡ]

4. *they*   [ðeɪ]

5. *soft*   [sɑft]

6. *tongue*   [tʌŋ]

7. *splash*   [splæʃ]

8. *squirrel*   [skwɝɫ]

9. *buzz*   [bʌz]

10. *caught*   [kɑt]

11. *sign*   [saɪn]

12. *who*   [hu]

10–7. Single-Syllable Words: 7

1. *use* [juz]

2. *vine* [va͡ɪn]

3. *sixths* [sɪkθs]

4. *treat* [tɹit]

5. *cloth* [klɑθ]

6. *fair* [fɛ͡ɚ]

7. *cut* [kʌt]

8. *day* [de͡ɪ]

9. *chin* [t͡ʃɪn]

10. *egg* [ɛg]

11. *the* [ðʌ]

12. *five* [fa͡ɪv]

10–8. Single-Syllable Words: 8

1. *age*   [e͡ɪd͡ʒ]

2. *camp*   [kæmp]

3. *good*   [ɡʊd]

4. *bill*   [bɪɫ]

5. *not*   [nɑt]

6. *razed*   [ɹe͡ɪzd]

7. *fun*   [fʌn]

8. *breath*   [bɹɛθ]

9. *seen*   [sin]

10. *tough*   [tʌf]

11. *threw*   [θɹu]

12. *key*   [ki]

10–9. Single-Syllable Words: 9

1. *sick*   [sɪk]

2. *glass*   [ɡlæs]

3. *shop*   [ʃɑp]

4. *groove* [ɡɹuv]

5. *hat*   [hæt]

6. *he*   [hi]

7. *in*   [ɪn]

8. *jazz*   [d͡ʒæz]

9. *kite*   [ka͡ɪt]

10. *straw* [stɹɑ]

11. *wake*   [we͡ɪk]

12. *tie*   [ta͡ɪ]

10–10. Single-Syllable Words: 10

1. *lose*   [luz]

2. *miss*   [mɪs]

3. *name*   [neɪm]

4. *bait*   [beɪt]

5. *cat*   [kæt]

6. *pill*   [pɪɫ]

7. *nice*   [naɪs]

8. *crush*   [kɹʌʃ]

9. *each*   [itʃ]

10. *this*   [ðɪs]

11. *staff*   [stæf]

12. *yes*   [jɛs]

10–11. Single-Syllable Words: 11

1. *hopped*   [hɑpt]

2. *oath*   [o͡ʊθ]

3. *pack*   [pæk]

4. *gifts*   [gɪfts]

5. *robe*   [ɹo͡ʊb]

6. *pry*   [pɹa͡ɪ]

7. *push*   [pʊʃ]

8. *bath*   [bæθ]

9. *geese*   [gis]

10. *read*   [ɹid]

11. *time*   [ta͡ɪm]

12. *rock*   [ɹɑk]

10–12. Single-Syllable Words: 12

1. *dwarf*   [dwɔɚf]

2. *see*   [si]

3. *ghost*   [go͡ʊst]

4. *leaf*   [lif]

5. *chain*   [t͡ʃe͡ɪn]

6. *lift*   [lɪft]

7. *rope*   [ɹo͡ʊp]

8. *which*   [wɪt͡ʃ]

9. *vine*   [va͡ɪn]

10. *date*   [de͡ɪt]

11. *sun*   [sʌn]

12. *team*   [tim]

10–13. Single-Syllable Words: 13

1. *strength*   [stɹɛŋkθ]

2. *that*   [ðæt]

3. *might*   [ma͡ɪt]

4. *wish*   [wɪʃ]

5. *cough*   [kɑf] – [kɔf]

6. *maps*   [mæps]

7. *cute*   [kjut]

8. *did*   [dɪd]

9. *nest*   [nɛst]

10. *this*   [ðɪs]

11. *knee*   [ni]

12. *threat*   [θɹɛt]

10–14. Multisyllabic Words: 1

1. *giant* [ˈd͡ʒaɪ.ənt]

2. *nephew* [ˈnɛ.fju]

3. *rather* [ˈɹæ.ðɚ]

4. *fishing* [ˈfɪ.ʃɪŋ]

5. *backache* [ˈbæ.ke͡ɪk]

6. *about* [əˈba͡ʊt]

7. *giggling* [ˈgɪ.gə.lɪŋ]

8. *jacket* [ˈd͡ʒæ.kət]

9. *kangaroo* [kæŋ.gəˈɹu]

10. *recent* [ˈɹi.sənt]

11. *adore* [əˈd͡ɔɚ]

12. *singer* [ˈsɪŋ.ɚ]

10–15. Multisyllabic Words: 2

1. *bacon*   [ˈbeɪ.kən]

2. *hammer*   [ˈhæ.mɚ]

3. *summer*   [ˈsʌ.mɚ]

4. *royal*   [ˈɹɔɪ.jəɫ]

5. *behold*   [bə.ˈhoʊɫd]

6. *advantage* [æd.ˈvæn.tədʒ]

7. *hanger*   [ˈhæŋ.ɚ]

8. *bachelor*   [ˈbætʃ.lɚ]

9. *kitchen*   [ˈkɪ.tʃən]

10. *calming*   [ˈkɔɫ.mɪŋ] – [ˈkɑɫ.mɪŋ]

11. *lodges*   [ˈlɑ.dʒəz]

12. *again*   [ə.ˈgɛn]

10–16. Multisyllabic Words: 3

1. *higher*   [ˈhaɪ.ɚ]

2. *bother*   [ˈbɑ.ðɚ]

3. *mahogany*   [mə.ˈhɑ.gə.ni]

4. *unit*   [ˈju.nət]

5. *ginger*   [ˈd͡ʒɪn.d͡ʒɚ]

6. *collage*   [kə.ˈlɑʒ]

7. *terrible*   [ˈtɛɚ.ə.bəɫ]

8. *agitate*   [ˈæ.d͡ʒə.teɪt]

9. *story*   [ˈstɔɚ.i]

10. *casual*   [ˈkæ.ʒu.əɫ]

11. *otter*   [ˈɑ.ɾɚ]

12. *number*   [ˈnʌm.bɚ]

10–17. Multisyllabic Words: 4

1. *along*   [ə.ˈlɔŋ] – [ə.ˈlɑŋ]

2. *music*   [ˈmju.zɪk]

3. *vision*   [ˈvɪ.ʒən]

4. *city*   [ˈsɪ.ɾi]

5. *beacon*   [ˈbi.kən]

6. *office*   [ˈɑ.fɪs]

7. *anger*   [ˈæŋ.gɚ]

8. *dizzy*   [ˈdɪ.zi]

9. *blanket*   [ˈblæŋ.kət]

10. *October*   [ɑk.ˈtoʊ.bɚ]

11. *anyhow*   [ˈɛ.ni.haʊ]

12. *coughing* [ˈkɑ.fɪŋ] – [ˈkɔ.fɪŋ]

10–18. Multisyllabic Words: 5

1. *banana*   [bə.ˈnæ.nə]

2. *occasion*   [ə.ˈkeɪ.ʒən]

3. *peaches*   [ˈpi.t͡ʃəz]

4. *carrot*   [ˈkɛɚ.ət]

5. *before*   [bə.ˈfɔɚ]

6. *eerie*   [ˈɪɚ.i]

7. *anything*   [ˈɛ.ni.θɪŋ]

8. *easy*   [ˈi.zi]

9. *somebody*   [ˈsʌm.bə.ɹi]

10. *either*   [ˈaɪ.ðɚ]

11. *ribbon*   [ˈɹɪ.bən]

12. *pretty*   [ˈpɹɪ.ɹi]

10–19. Multisyllabic Words: 6

1. *aphasia*   [ə.ˈfeɪ.ʒə]

2. *zodiac*   [ˈzoʊ.ɹi.æk]

3. *profit*   [ˈpɹɑ.fɪt]

4. *usual*   [ˈju.ʒu.əɫ]

5. *ripen*   [ˈɹaɪ.pən]

6. *family*   [ˈfæ.mə.li]

7. *stopping*   [ˈstɑ.pɪŋ]

8. *toothbrush*   [ˈtuθ.bɹəʃ]

9. *coffee*   [ˈkɑ.fi]

10. *single*   [ˈsɪŋ.gəɫ]

11. *weather*   [ˈwɛ.ðɚ]

12. *potato*   [pə.ˈteɪ.ɹoʊ]

10–20. Multisyllabic Words: 7

1. envious [ˈɛn.vi.əs]

2. bucket [ˈbʌ.kɪt]

3. stocking [ˈstɑ.kɪŋ]

4. burrito [bɚ.ˈɹi.ɾoʊ]

5. fasten [ˈfæ.sɪn]

6. prestige [pɹɛs.ˈtiʒ]

7. visit [ˈvɪ.zət]

8. feather [ˈfɛ.ðɚ]

9. ashamed [ə.ˈʃeɪmd]

10. lesson [ˈlɛ.sən]

11. fashion [ˈfæ.ʃən]

12. gentle [ˈd͡ʒɛn.təɫ]

10–21. Multisyllabic Words: 8

1. *value*   ['væɫ.ju]

2. *begin*   [bə.ˈɡɪn]

3. *peanut*   [ˈpi.nət]

4. *Athens*   [ˈæ.θɪnz]

5. *magic*   [ˈmæ.d͡ʒɪk]

6. *orange*   [ˈɔɚ.ənd͡ʒ]

7. *possible*   [ˈpɑ.sə.bəɫ]

8. *servant*   [ˈsɚ.vənt]

9. *widen*   [ˈwaɪ.ɹən]

10. *ego*   [ˈi.ɡo͡ʊ]

11. *wealthy*   [ˈwɛɫ.θi]

12. *treasure*   [ˈtɹɛ.ʒɚ]

10–22. Multisyllabic Words: 9

1. *virtue*   [ˈvɝ.t͡ʃu]

2. *basin*   [ˈbe͡ɪ.sɪn]

3. *voyage*   [ˈvɔ͡ɪ.əd͡ʒ]

4. *breathy*   [ˈbɹɛ.θi]

5. *cathedral*   [kə.ˈθi.dɹəɫ]

6. *yellow*   [ˈjɛ.lo͡ʊ]

7. *believe*   [bə.ˈliv]

8. *wishes*   [ˈwɪ.ʃəz]

9. *rehearse*   [ɹi.ˈhɝs]

10. *dollar*   [ˈdɑ.lɚ]

11. *earthquake*   [ˈɝθ.kwe͡ɪk]

12. *father*   [ˈfɑ.ðɚ]

10–23. Multisyllabic Words: 10

1. *happy*   [ˈhæ.pi]

2. *jelly*   [ˈd͡ʒɛ.li]

3. *kitten*   [ˈkɪ.ʔən]

4. *loyal*   [ˈlɔɪ.əɫ]

5. *mother*   [ˈmʌ.ðɚ]

6. *nation*   [ˈneɪ.ʃən]

7. *obvious*   [ˈɑb.vi.əs]

8. *bigger*   [ˈbɪ.gɚ]

9. *oppose*   [ə.ˈpoʊz]

10. *pebble*   [ˈpɛ.bəɫ]

11. *dozen*   [ˈdʌ.zɪn]

12. *camouflage* [ˈkæ.mə.flɑʒ]

10–24. Short Phrases: 1

1. *black cat*   [blæk kæt]

2. *hot water*   [hɑʔ ˈwɑ.ɾɚ]

3. *poster board*   [ˈpoʊs.tɚ bɔɚd]

4. *yellow ladder*   [ˈjɛ.loʊ ˈlæ.ɾɚ]

5. *purple paint*   [ˈpɝ.pəł peɪnt]

6. *icy pavement*   [ˈaɪ.si ˈpeɪv.mɛnt]

7. *galloping horse*   [ˈgæ.lə.pɪŋ hɔɚs]

8. *take care*   [teɪk kɛɚ]

9. *early riser*   [ˈɝ.li ˈɹaɪ.zɚ]

10. *crowded buses*   [ˈkɹaʊ.ɾɪd ˈbʌ.sɪz]

11. *phonetic transcription*   [fə.ˈnɛ.ɾɪk tɹæn.ˈskɹɪp.ʃən]

12. *communication disorder*   [kə.mju.nɪ.ˈkeɪ.ʃən dɪ.ˈsɔɚ.ɾɚ]

10–25. Short Phrases: 2

1. *rotating disks*   [ˈɹoʊ.teɪ.ɾɪŋ dɪsks]

2. *devoted students*   [dɪ.ˈvoʊ.ɾəd ˈstu.ɹənts]

3. *eager beaver*   [ˈi.gɚ ˈbi.vɚ]

4. *auditory processing*   [ˈɔ.ɾɪ.tɔɚ.i ˈpɹɑ.sɛ.sɪŋ] – [ˈɑ.ɾɪ.tɔɚ.i ˈpɹɑ.sɛ.sɪŋ]

5. *migraine headache*   [ˈmaɪ.gɹeɪn ˈhɛ.deɪk]

6. *bouncing baby*   [ˈbaʊn.sɪŋ ˈbeɪbi]

7. *chocolate cheesecake*   [ˈt͡ʃak.lɛt ˈt͡ʃiz.keɪk]

8. *Caribbean cruise*   [kə.ˈɹɪ.bi.ɪn kɹuz]

9. *destroyed building*   [dɪs.ˈtɹɔɪd ˈbɪɫ.dɪŋ]

10. *one toothbrush*   [wən ˈtuθ.bɹəʃ]

11. *measuring cups*   [ˈmɛ.ʒɚ.ɪŋ kʌps]

12. *happy birthday*   [ˈhæ.pi ˈbɝθ.deɪ]

10–26. Longer Phrases: 1

1. *fabulous mosaic*   ['fæb.jə.lɪs mo͡ʊ.'ze͡ɪ.ɪk]

2. *talking chatterbox*   ['tɔ.kɪŋ 't͡ʃæ.ɾɚ.bɑks] – ['tɑ.kɪŋ 't͡ʃæ.ɾɚ.bɑks]

3. *playing the harp*   [ple͡ɪ.ɪŋ ðə hɑɚ.p]

4. *elephants in pajamas*   ['ɛ.lɪ.fɪnts ɪn pə.'d͡ʒæ.məz]

5. *fudge mint Oreos*   [fʌd͡ʒ mɪnt 'ɔɚ.i.o͡ʊz]

6. *azure ocean blue*   ['æ.ʒɚ 'o͡ʊ.ʃən blu]

7. *ladies and gentlemen*   ['le͡ɪ.ɾiz ænd 'd͡ʒɛn.təɫ.mɪn]

8. *bagels or strudel*   ['be͡ɪ.gəɫz ɔɚ 'stɹu.ɾəɫ]

9. *going skiing*   [a͡ɪm 'go͡ʊ.ɪŋ 'ski.ɹŋ]

10. *ticket's booked*   ['tɪ.kəts bʊkt]

11. *person of wealth*   ['pɝ.sən əv wɛɫθ]

12. *cheddar cheese quesadillas* ['t͡ʃɛ.ɾɚ t͡ʃiz 'ke͡ɪ.sə.ɾi.əz]

10–27. Longer Phrases: 2

1. *brown paper packages*   [bɹaʊn 'peɪ.pɚ 'pæ.kə.d͡ʒɪz]

2. *gigantic eighteen wheeler*   [d͡ʒaɪ.'gæn.tɪk 'eɪ.tin 'wi.lɚ]

3. *Californian abstract artist*   ['kæ.lɪ.fɔ͡ɚ.njən 'æb.stɹækt 'a͡ɚ.ɹɪst]

4. *professor of audiology*   [pɹə.'fɛ.sɚ əv ɔ.ɹi.'a.lə.d͡ʒi] – [pɹə.'fɛ.sɚ əv a.ɹi.'a.lə.d͡ʒi]

5. *sprint up the hill*   [spɹɪnt əp ðə hɪɫ]

6. *colorful impressionist painting*   ['kʌ.lɚ.fʊɫ ɪm.'pɹɛ.ʃə.nɪst 'pe͡ɪn.tɪŋ]

7. *flexible Olympic gymnast*   ['flɛk.sɪ.bəɫ ə.'lɪm.pɪk 'd͡ʒɪm.nɪst]

8. *bright blossoming sunflower*   [bɹaɪt 'bla.sə.mɪŋ 'sʌn.fla͡ʊɚ]

9. *triangles, squares, rectangles*   ['tɹa͡ɪ.æŋ.gəɫz, skwɛ͡ɚz, 'ɹɛk.tæŋ.gəɫz]

10. *remembering childhood daydreams*   [ɹi.'mɛm.bɚ.ɪŋ 't͡ʃaɪɫd.hʊd 'de͡ɪ.dɹimz]

11. *rambunctious kindergarteners*   [ɹæm.'bʌŋk.ʃɪs 'kɪn.dɚ.ga͡ɚd.nɚz]

12. *delicious huckleberry pie*   [də.'lɪ.ʃɪs 'hʌ.kəɫ.bɛ͡ɚ.i pa͡ɪ]

10–28. Sentences: 1

1. *Please fasten your seatbelts.*
[pliz 'fæ.sɪn jɔɚ 'sit.bɛɬts]

2. *I'd like to order the vegetable souffle.*
[aɪd laɪk tu 'ɔɚ.rɚ ðə 'vɛdʒ.tə.bʊɬ su.'fleɪ]

3. *Five o'clock is rush hour.*
['faɪ.v ə.klɑk ɪz ɹʌʃ aʊɚ]

4. *She is certain it's not pouring.*
[ʃi ɪz 'sɝ.tɪn ɪts nɑt 'pɔɚ.ɪŋ]

5. *My favorite movie is Jurassic Park.*
[maɪ 'feɪv.ɹɪt 'mu.vi ɪz dʒə.'ɹæ.sɪk pɑɚk]

6. *She went to her high school reunion.*
[ʃi wɛnt tu hɝ 'haɪ skuɬ ɹi.'jun.jən]

7. *He wore a tuxedo with shiny black shoes.*
[hi wɔɚ eɪ tək.'si.ɹoʊ wɪθ 'ʃaɪ.ni blæk ʃuz]

8. *The garden is overflowing with shrubs and bushes.*
[ðə 'gɑɚ.ɹɪn ɪz oʊ.vɚ.'floʊ.ɪŋ wɪθ ʃɹʌbz ænd bʊ.ʃəz]

9. *Spaghetti is a delicious meal.*
[spə.'gɛ.ɹi ɪz eɪ di.'lɪ.ʃəs miɬ]

10. *Don't be noisy or you'll get in trouble.*
[doʊnt bi 'nɔɪ.zi ɔɚ juɬ gɛt ɪn 'tɹʌ.bəɬ]

11. *Leopard print is back in fashion.*
['lɛ.pɚd pɹɪnt ɪz bæk ɪn 'fæ.ʃən]

12. *Turn up the stereo, so I can hear the music.*
[tɝn əp ðə 'stɛɚ.i.oʊ soʊ aɪ kæn hɪɚ ðə 'mju.zɪk]

10–29. Sentences: 2

1. *Report the theft to the state police.*
   [ɹiˈpɔɚt ðə θɛft tu ðə steɪt pəˈlis]

2. *Study hard and you will succeed.*
   [ˈstʌɾi hɑɚd ænd ju wɪɫ səkˈsid]

3. *He plays the electric guitar.*
   [hi pleɪz ðə əˈlɛk.tɹɪk gɪˈtɑɚ]

4. *My friend sews floral pillowcases.*
   [maɪ fɹɛnd soʊz ˈflɔɚ.əɫ ˈpɪ.loʊ ˈkeɪ.sɪz]

5. *The record player has broken again.*
   [ðə ˈɹɛ.kɚd ˈpleɪ.ɚ hæz ˈbɹoʊ.kɪn əˈgɛn]

6. *Store leftovers in plastic containers.*
   [stɔɚ ˈlɛf.toʊ.vɚz ɪn ˈplæ.stɪk kənˈteɪ.nɚz]

7. *Stop talking while I'm watching the television.*
   [stɑp ˈtɔ.kɪŋ waɪɫ aɪm ˈwa.tʃɪŋ ðə ˈtɛ.lə.vɪ.ʒən] – [stɑp ˈta.kɪŋ waɪɫ aɪm ˈwa.tʃɪŋ ðə ˈtɛ.lə.vɪ.ʒən]

8. *Consonants are either voiced or voiceless.*
   [ˈkan.sə.nɪnts ɑɚ ˈi.ðɚ vɔɪst ɔɚ ˈvɔɪs.lɛs]

9. *Chocolate brownies with marshmallow sauce taste good.*
   [ˈtʃɔ.klɛt ˈbɹaʊ.niz wɪθ ˈmɑɚʃ.mɛ.loʊ sas teɪst gʊd] –
   [ˈtʃɑ.klɛt ˈbɹaʊ.niz wɪθ ˈmɑɚʃ.mɛ.loʊ sas teɪst gʊd]

10. *Be nice to all the teacher's assistants.*
    [bi naɪs tu aɫ ðə ˈti. tʃɚz əˈsɪ.stɪnts]

11. *Can I borrow a pencil?*
    [kæn aɪ ˈbɑɚ.oʊ ə ˈpɛn.səɫ]

12. *My chores take hours to finish.*
    [maɪ tʃɔɚz teɪk aʊɚz tu ˈfɪ.nɪʃ]

10–30. Sentences: 3

1. *The flowers are pretty.*
   [ðə 'flaʊ.wɚz ɑɚ 'pɹɪ.ɾi]

2. *There is a bird in that tree.*
   [ðɛɚ ɪz ə bɝd ɪn ðæt tɹi]

3. *The child's singing is lovely.*
   [ðə t͡ʃaɪɫdz 'sɪ.ŋɪŋ ɪz 'lʌv.li]

4. *Raindrops are falling from the sky.*
   ['ɹeɪn.dɹɑps ɑɚ 'fɑ.lɪŋ fɹəm ðə skaɪ]

5. *My sister is a judge on the Supreme Court.*
   [maɪ 'sɪs.tɚ ɪz ə d͡ʒʌd͡ʒ ɑn ðə sə.'prim kɔɚt]

6. *Did you study for the test?*
   [dɪd ju 'stʌ.ɾi fɔɚ ðə tɛst]

7. *In the winter, I like to ski with my friends and family.*
   [ɪn ðə 'wɪn.tɚ aɪ laɪk tu ski wɪθ maɪ fɹɛndz ænd 'fæm.li]

8. *Will you come to my birthday party on Friday?*
   [wɪl ju kəm tu maɪ 'bɝθ.deɪ 'pɑɚ.ɾi ɑn 'fɹaɪ.deɪ]

9. *He is the fastest racer.*
   [hi ɪz ðə 'fæ.stɪst 'ɹeɪ.sɚ]

10. *I will meet you there in one hour to work on the group project.*
    [aɪ wɪɫ mit ju ðɛɚ ɪn wʌn aʊɚ tə wɚk ɑn ðə gɹup 'pɹɑ. d͡ʒɛkt]

11. *She sells seashells by the seashore.*
    [ʃi sɛɫz 'si.ʃɛɫz baɪ ðə 'si.ʃɔɚ]

12. *I scream, you scream, we all scream for ice cream.*
    [aɪ skɹim ju skɹim wi ɑɫ skɹim fɔɚ 'aɪs.kɹim]

10–31. Sentences: 4

1. *Put the books away.*
   [pʊt ðə bʊks ə.ˈweɪ]

2. *Two young boys are looking for their toys.*
   [tu jʌŋ bɔɪz ɑ˞ ˈlʊ.kɪŋ fɔ˞ ðɛɚ tɔɪz]

3. *I love the music on this tour.*
   [aɪ lʌv ðə ˈmju.zɪk ɑn ðɪs tʊɚ]

4. *Wish upon a star.*
   [wɪʃ ə.ˈpɑn ə stɑɚ]

5. *Let's go see a movie.*
   [lɛts goʊ si ə ˈmu.vi]

6. *Where are you from?*
   [wɛɚ ɑ˞ ju fɹʌm]

7. *I've heard so much about you.*
   [aɪv hɝd soʊ mʌtʃ ə.ˈbaʊt ju]

8. *The rabbit got out of his cage and now he is missing.*
   [ðə ˈɹæ.bət gɑt aʊt ʌv hɪz keɪdʒ ænd naʊ hi ɪz ˈmɪ.sɪŋ]

9. *It's so good to see you again.*
   [ɪts soʊ gʊd tu si ju ə.ˈgɛn]

10. *Tourists like to go whale watching when they visit the coast.*
    [ˈtʊɚ.ɪsts laɪk tu goʊ weɪɫ ˈwɑ.tʃɪŋ wɛn ðeɪ ˈvɪ.zɪt ðə koʊst]

11. *What time does the bus arrive?*
    [wət taɪm dəz ðə bʌs ə.ˈɹaɪv]

12. *Thank you for giving me a ride to the airport in the middle of the night.*
    [θæŋk ju fɔ˞ ˈgɪ.vɪŋ mi ə ɹaɪd tu ðə ˈɛɚ.pɔɚt ɪn ðə ˈmɪ.ɹəɫ əv ðə naɪt]

10–32. Sentences: 5

1. *It is important to measure ingredients when baking.*
   [ɪt ɪz ɪm.ˈpɔɚ.ɾənt tu ˈmɛ.ʒɚ ɪŋ.ˈɡɹi.ɾi.ɪnts wɛn ˈbeɪ.kɪŋ]

2. *There are a lot of fish swimming upstream this time of year.*
   [ðɛɚ ɑɚ ə lɑt ʌv fɪʃ ˈswɪ.mɪŋ ˈʌp.stɹim ðɪs taɪm əv jɪɚ]

3. *Where is the nearest hospital?*
   [wɛɚ ɪz ðə nɪɚ.əst ˈhɑ.spɪ.təɫ

4. *Do not touch service dogs when they are working.*
   [du nɑt tʌtʃ ˈsɝ.vɪs dɑgz wɛn ðeɪ ɑɚ ˈwɝ.kɪŋ] – [du nɑt tʌtʃ ˈsɝ.vɪs dɔgz wɛn ðeɪ ɑɚ ˈwɝ.kɪŋ]

5. *She can read and write very well for her age.*
   [ʃi kæn ɹid ænd ɹaɪt ˈvɛɚ.i wɛɫ fɔɚ hɚ eɪdʒ]

6. *Kids often forget their jackets at school.*
   [kɪdz ˈɔf.tɛn fɔɚ.ˈgɛt ðɛɚ ˈdʒæ.kɪts æt skuɫ]

7. *The rose garden is growing nicely this year.*
   [ðə ɹoʊz ˈgɑɚ.ɾɛn ɪz ˈgɹoʊ.ɪŋ ˈnaɪs.li ðɪs jɪɚ]

8. *His dream is to be a homeowner.*
   [hɪz dɹim ɪz tu bi ə ˈhoʊ.moʊ.nɚ]

9. *You will need a bow and arrows for your first archery lesson.*
   [ju wɪɫ nid ə boʊ ænd ˈɛɚ.oʊz fɔɚ jɚ fɝst ˈɑɚ.tʃɚ.i ˈlɛ.sən]

10. *Jack loves to go camping during spring break.*
    [dʒæk lʌvz tu goʊ ˈkæm.pɪŋ ˈdɚ.ɪŋ spɹɪŋ bɹeɪk]

11. *She is graduating from high school in June.*
    [ʃi ɪz ˈgɹæ.dʒu.weɪ.ɾɪŋ frəm ˈhaɪ skuɫ ɪn dʒun]

12. *My cousin will be visiting us in the summer.*
    [maɪ ˈkʌ.zən wɪɫ bi ˈvɪ.zə.ɾɪŋ ʌs ɪn ðə ˈsʌ.mɚ]